Doctoring Data

*How to sort out medical advice
from medical nonsense*

Dr Malcolm Kendrick

Published by Columbus Publishing Ltd 2014
www.columbuspublishing.co.uk

ISBN 978-1-907797-46-0
Rev 20150202

A CIP record of this book is available from the British Library.

Cover design by Lewis Kokoc

Typesetting by Raffaele Bolelli Gallevi

Brand and product names are trademarks or registered trademarks
of their respective owners.

The content of this book is intended to inform, entertain and provoke your thinking. This is not intended as medical advice. It may, however, make you question current medical and nutritional advice. That's your choice. It's your life and health in your hands. Neither the author nor the publisher can be held responsible or liable for any loss or claim arising from the use, or misuse, of the content of this book.

COLUMBUS PUBLISHING

"If people let the government decide what foods they eat and what medicines they take, their bodies will soon be in as sorry a state as are the souls who live under tyranny."

Thomas Jefferson (1743 - 1826)

Reviews for Doctoring Data

"A rollicking rant about everything that is suspect in modern medicine."
Professor Iona Heath, former president of the Royal College of General Practitioners

"Dr Kendrick shares with the reader his wit, humor and laser-sharp insights to expose the misinformation underlying accepted health guidelines. His book is an exposé on a broad range of flawed research and treatments, including the unnecessary and unhealthy reduction of cholesterol with statins, the dubious effectiveness of influenza treatment with Tamiflu and the demonization of saturated fat. Dr Kendrick has a unique talent to explain the conceptual and methodological flaws in a broad range of scientific studies which is of value to all clinicians, and is presented at a level which can be understood by laypeople. This book is a must read for anyone interested in becoming aware of how deception and financial conflict interest have dominated current health guidelines and treatment recommendations."
David Diamond, Ph.D. Departments of Psychology, Molecular Pharmacology and Physiology, University of South Florida and Medical Research Service, Tampa Veterans Hospital

"In this witty exposé, Dr Malcolm Kendrick daringly prises open paradoxes, trade secrets and shoddy statistics that lie behind so much of modern medicine.
"His highly entertaining and informative book undermines accepted wisdom of Britain's biggest health risks and shines a spotlight onto how persuasive and profit hungry drug companies have brought harmful and potentially unproven treatments to market.
"Dr Kendrick is a maverick but his disturbing assertions are worryingly backed by strong evidence."
Lucy Johnston. Health and social affairs editor, *The Express*

"Dr Malcolm Kendrick will challenge you to question everything you've ever been told about science from the media, from the so-called 'experts' and those organizations with vested interests.

"As an investigative journalist, I've always believed that a fact is a fact, but now I question whether a 'fact' is also the 'truth'. Dr Kendrick reveals much of what we've been told by trusted health authorities has been influenced in some way, either by poor quality evidence or industry sponsorship, or both. Most concerning is that these issues affect the very guidelines that influence doctors' prescribing habits and the distribution of health advice.

"Scientific research is supposed to encourage critical thinking but as Kendrick points out time and time again, those who 'rock the boat' and challenge the establishment, are often persecuted - either with threats to funding, to their careers and/or their reputations.

"As a former scientist, there were moments in this book where I felt utterly frustrated with my former profession. Cognitive dissonance is widespread in an environment where there is competition for laboratory funding and the publication of results in prestigious journals. With most of the clinical drug trials nowadays being funded by the manufacturers who directly profit from drug sales, it's no wonder we have biased science that accentuates the benefits and underplays the risks. Sound cynical? I encourage you to read the book and make up your own mind.

"This book promises to take you on a journey that will both frustrate and enthrall you."

Dr Maryanne Demasi, Ph.D. Producer/Investigative reporter, ABC TV Australia

"Malcolm Kendrick is the Mark Twain of medical writers, wielding his own pen warmed up in hell – hell, in this case, being a medical system designed to persuade doctors that nearly everyone with a pulse is abnormal and in need of treatment. In fact, I can summarize Kendrick's Doctoring Data by paraphrasing Twain himself: 'If your doctor doesn't read the medical literature, he is uninformed. If he does read the medical literature, he is misinformed.'

"Your doctor can afford to be misinformed. You cannot - that is, unless you don't mind being diagnosed with a previously unknown 'disease' ... which was discovered just in time to coincide with development of a new wonder drug ... which was approved based on suspicious data ... from a study designed and run by the drug-maker ...which paid key opinion leaders to sit on a government committee that wrote the treatment guidelines ... which instruct your doctor to prescribe the new wonder drug ... which produces nasty side-effects ... which must be treated with more wonder drugs.

"Kendrick pulls back the curtains and invites the reader to understand how this system works (or more correctly, doesn't work), serving as a tour guide who *happens to be as laugh-out-loud funny as he is informative. For your own protection, I suggest you take the tour."*

Tom Naughton, health blogger and writer/director of the documentary
Fat Head: you've been fed a load of bologna

"Doctoring Data is the perfect antidote to the medical establishment's recycled dogma. Dr Malcolm Kendrick is one of the sharpest, best informed, most provocative challengers of received medical wisdom. His engagingly irreverent and witty insights into how scientific 'fact' and 'consensus' is manufactured are electrifying. Whether he is turning his attention to drug trials, or to bariatric surgery, everything Dr Kendrick writes is worth reading."

Joanna Blythman, award-winning journalist and author of
Shopped, What To Eat, and *Bad Food Britain*

"'The only end of writing,' said Samuel Johnson, 'is to enable the reader better to enjoy life, or better to endure it.' The great man would clearly have treasured every page of Doctoring Data.

"Kendrick's latest work is the ultimate exposé on the modern medical establishment.

"Every reader stands to change their lives forever after reading this book. If that fact does not make you seek out a copy then stay smiling in the dark. Ignorance is bliss, until it kills you."

Justin Stoneman, Journalist and broadcaster

"If every doctor and scientist had as much honesty, integrity and quick wit as Dr Kendrick then we would not be in such a sorry state of affairs. If you want to become a better doctor or scientist then you need to read this book."

Sam Feltham, Author of *Slimology* & Founder of *Smash The Fat*

"Kendrick is witty, hard-hitting, and irreverent, as he illuminates some of the egregious scientific practices that have been used to underpin many of our misguided health recommendations today. He makes complex scientific subjects simple for the average reader - like what's wrong with linear modeling? His investigation into corporations that finance scientists - 'the hand that feeds' - is a special treat."

Nina Teicholz, author of *The Big Fat Surprise: Why Butter, Meat & Cheese Belong in a Healthy Diet*

"Most of us witness the news every day with increasingly slack-jawed amazement. 'Do these people think we're idiots?' we commonly shout at the TV, newspa-

per and websites, which is a peculiarly silly waste of time and can get you arrested in public libraries. But for those of us for whom this is a way of life, Dr Malcolm Kendrick's book Doctoring Data is a welcome friend.

"Ever had the feeling that your doctor is a fool? Yeah, me too. Ever had the feeling they're pushing you drugs you don't need for illnesses you don't have? Yeah, me too. Ever get the feeling that they're passing off guesswork, marketing ploys and downright corrupt data as fact? Yeah, me too.

"Kendrick tackles all of these issues and more head on and lays bare how, when it comes to medical, health and food matters, we are being fed ignorance as though it is intelligence and misinformation as though it is truth. He rationally exposes the innate corruption that lies at the heart of the industries which cream up big profits on the back of ill people and even bigger profits from people whom they seek to define as ill but who are perfectly healthy.

"He shows how a white coat and some letters after your name is used to con us into thinking there is more efficacy and evidence to health claims than there is and better still, he does this with great humour, because frankly, if you didn't laugh about these scandals, you'd cry.

John Nicholson, Novelist, Writer, Columnist

"We have become used to thinking as a cohort, and believing that our leaders, the great and the good, will have found us the right collective answers.

"While reading this book, I call upon individuals to think, to put themselves in the jury box, evaluate the evidence and work out the probable truth for any question, statement or allegation.

"I believe Kendrick's book The Great Cholesterol Con is essential reading for all people and not just all health professionals in the Western World, where we have medicated normality. When most of the evidence is in front of you, it is possible to reach a reasonable conclusion and decide your own way forward.

"This new book Doctoring Data addresses several areas where our collective wisdom has been manipulated and we have been taught to think in an unhelpful and sometimes harmful way. Read it and evaluate it. Read it and decide what you believe."

Dr Joanne McCormack GP Warrington UK

"We all think that evidence-based medicine is a good idea. But how many of us really understand how the evidence is skewed to serve financial, corporate or personal interests? Even if we are generally aware of the extent to which this happens, how can we precisely determine when the 'evidence' is reliable and when it has been spun all out of proportion? Dr Kendrick has been studying this for three *decades and after reading his book, I guarantee that you will never look at health news or published research in the same way again.*

"Doctoring Data lifts the veil of deception often surrounding the reporting of medical research. You should read it if you have even the remotest interest in your own health or the health of someone else. Every health journalist should also read this book - if they did, we would immediately see a drastic improvement in the way that medical studies are reported.

"Now that almost all of the medical research is funded, conducted, and reported by corporations with vested interests, it is essential that patients and future patients become savvy consumers of medicines and perhaps more importantly, the medical data. Understanding medical research might seem daunting, however, Dr Kendrick has managed to cover all of the important aspects in this very readable book.

"Reading the book, I felt that the seriousness of the topics covered was palpable. However, at the same time, Dr Kendrick has skillfully called upon his famous dry sense of humour to highly entertain the reader along the way.

"It is important to note that Dr Kendrick does not tell you what you should do. Throughout the book he reminds the reader that each of us should make informed personal decisions about medicines and other health issues. Probably the most powerful thing about this book is that it has the potential to completely transform patient-doctor interactions for the better. Dr Kendrick has provided an extremely powerful tool for people who have a desire to take personal responsibility for their own health.

Justin Smith, Producer/Director: *$TATIN NATION*

"Doctoring Data confirms Mark Twain's assertion that 'Figures don't lie but liars can figure', and that 'There are lies, damned lies and statistics.' The first law of statistics is that given enough statistics, you can prove anything. The second is that if the statistics don't support your theory, you need more statistics.

"This book supports the research of John Ionnadis, which concluded that '41% of the 49 most influential research studies in medicine have been convincingly shown to be wrong or significantly exaggerated', and that that up to 90% of medical publications doctors rely on is flawed. Some of the reasons for this are that so many studies are funded by Big Pharma, which is increasingly devoted to converting healthy people into paying patients by hyping trivial complaints into diseases requiring prescription drugs or by inventing new diseases that may respond to an existing drug.

"Once a drug is approved by the FDA as safe, it can be prescribed for any condition. Pharmaceutical manufacturers also have significant clout on the pub-

lication process, since medical journals don't want to jeopardize their lucrative income from advertisements and reprints by including articles with unfavorable drug studies.

"This book shows how pharmacracy, disease mongering and medicalization of healthy people has transformed a profession devoted to healing into a trade or commercial enterprise where the goal is to increase profits. This includes making diseases out of a wide range of human behaviors from alcoholism and obesity to emotional disturbances and infertility, some of which have been elevated to public health problems that are then subject to government intervention.

"It should be required reading for practitioners and all medical students."

Paul J. Rosch, MD, FACP, Clinical Professor of Medicine and Psychiatry, New York Medical College. Chairman of the Board, The American Institute of Stress

"I haven't laughed this much since I first watched 'The Life of Brian'!"

Kate Jones, Sixth form critical thinking teacher

"Doctoring Data is a timely masterpiece- a clever, witty and devastating analysis of the facade of knowledge that sustains the current medical enthusiasm for overdiagnosis and overtreatment,and its devastating consequences for so many. Obligatory reading."

James Le Fanu, author of The Rise & Fall of Modern Medicine

Dr Kendrick does not write out of ego or arrogance. He writes because he has seen the truth and he finds that truth very disturbing. He writes as a general practitioner working in the front lines of modern medicine. He is not an ivory-tower academic; yet his grasp of science exceeds that of most such academics. He writes solely to empower the individual because he believes that "knowledge is power". Certainly I who live and breath science, have been empowered by the scientific knowledge I have gained from his writings.

Thank you Dr Kendrick. You have made a significant difference to my understanding.

Now we must insure that everyone in our profession and most especially those just entering it, be exposed to this empowering information. It is beyond important.

The future of our profession may just depend on our understanding why we believe as we do.

And why we are usually wrong.

Timothy Noakes OMS, MBChB, MD, DSc, PhD (hc), FACSM, (hc) FFSEM
Emeritus Professor, University of Cape Town, South Africa.

Thank You

Nikki, my wife, for having to listen to my ramblings over the years, and for helping me to see the wood for the trees.

Luke Kendrick, my son, for coming up with the title of this book and reminding me to keep my sense of humour.

My father, Bill Kendrick, for tearing pages out of textbooks when I was younger and announcing that 'this is complete rubbish.' This opened my eyes to the fact that, just because an 'expert' says something, that doesn't make it right, or true.

Uffe Ravnskov, founder of 'The International Network of Cholesterol Skeptics', a visionary, a man who seeks the truth, and an inspiration to many of us who battle against medical dogma.

My Daughter, Catriona Kendrick. She kept my enthusiasm for medicine alive by being so interested and keen on it, and then heading off to medical school.

Zoë Harcombe, for her bright enthusiasm, her encouragement of my ideas, and her tireless energy to expose nonsense in the world of medical research.

Doctoring Data

Contents

Let me tell you a story...

A good friend is a GP not far away from me, in a very affluent part of the Thames Valley, with patients who are not short of money. One, an elderly widow, was picked up by the MIGPs[i] after falling at home, and after being seen in Accident & Emergency (A&E), was referred to the falls clinic. She asked my friend whether she should go. *'Sure, why not?'* replied my friend.

A few weeks later, the elderly lady booked an appointment to see my friend. She attended surgery dressed as impeccably as ever. In her cut-glass voice, she said to my friend:

"This falls clinic nonsense. What the fuck is that about? Are people really paid to do this sort of thing? The blithering idiot asked me if I had any idea why I'd fallen over. I'm ninety-bloody-two, for goodness' sake. Given the amount of gin I drink, it'd be a bloody miracle if I didn't fall over!"

Hallelujah!

We need more patients like that.

This book is written for all gin-soaked 92 year olds the world over – although I am hoping that my target audience may be a bit wider than this. It might include gin-soaked men and women of all ages. Those who drink inferior spirits are also welcome. As for malt whisky drinkers... bless you all. You too are welcome. 'Ceud mìle fàilte.'

---

i MIGPs stands for 'Men In Green Pyjamas'. It is what doctors call paramedics when they are out of ear shot. And sometimes when they are in ear shot too. It is part of the banter that patients are mainly, blissfully, unaware of.

Introduction

"Everything I like is either illegal, immoral, or fattening."
Thomas Woolcot

It has become exceedingly difficult to enjoy life's simple pleasures. Lying in the sun... "Do *not* do that, or you will die of skin cancer." Eating a bacon sandwich... "You mad fool, the saturated fat in that will raise your cholesterol levels and you *will* die of heart disease." Putting salt on food... "That raises blood pressure and you will *die* of a heart attack or a stroke." Drinking an ice-cold gin and tonic after a hard day's work... "If you drink more than 15 units a week you risk dying of cancer and liver failure." Hey ho, what jolly fun.

At the same time we are being cajoled to undergo ever more screening tests to pick up the early stages of cancer and numerous other diseases. As if this were not enough, your GP will be haranguing you to have endless measurements of blood pressure, cholesterol, and blood sugar levels, to name but three. As if good health is only really possible through constant monitoring by the medical profession.

As for the elderly, it has become virtually impossible to find anyone taking fewer than four or five separate medications. One of my jobs is working in Intermediate Care where I help to look after elderly people, many of whom have suffered an injury or fracture of some sort. When patients enter this unit, the average number of medications taken is ten. That is ten different drugs, to be taken each and every day, some of them three or four times each day. I suppose it saves on buying food.

At the same time, the boundaries that define illness have narrowed inexorably. When I first graduated from medical school in 1981, a high cholesterol level was anything above 7.5 mmol/L. Over the years, this level has fallen and fallen to the point where a 'healthy' level is now 5.0 mmol/L. I suspect it will soon be 4.0 mmol/L. Anything above this figure, and you have an increased risk of heart disease – allegedly.

Considering that over 85% of the adult population in the western world has a cholesterol level higher than 5.0 mmol/L this is a quite amazing concept. I will admit that I have never been that brilliant at statistics. However, it seems to me that attempting to claim that more than 80% of people are at high risk of heart disease stretches the concept of 'average' to breaking point – and well beyond.

In much the same vein, a high blood pressure used to be something above 160/110 mmHg. It is now 140/90 mmHg – or even lower, depending on which guidelines you read. For those with diabetes, a raised level is anything above 120/85 mmHg. At the same time, the concept of 'pre-hypertension' is gaining ground. Here are some words of wisdom on pre-hypertension from *WebMD*:

"'There is increasing evidence of the relationship between an elevated blood pressure and future problems with heart attack and stroke. With each level of increase in pressure, you get increased risk,' he [Sheldon Sheps] tells WebMD.

"Consider these startling statistics. Starting as low as 115/75, the risk of heart attack and stroke doubles for every 20-point jump in systolic blood pressure or every 10-point rise in diastolic blood pressure.

"'We've also learned that people age 55 and older, who currently have normal blood pressure, have a 90% risk of developing high blood pressure down the road,' says Aram Chobanian, MD, Dean of Boston University School of Medicine, who chaired the guidelines committee."[1]

So, a high blood pressure is now anything above 115/75 mmHg. I bet that just cheered you up. In addition, for those of you who smugly believed that your blood pressure is still considered normal, it seems you have a 90% risk of developing high blood pressure in the end. You are merely temporarily well... earthling.

It seems we have very nearly reached the point where there really is no such thing as a normal blood pressure any more. We are all either hypertensive, pre-hypertensive, or will inevitably develop hypertension in the end... which may, or may not, mean exactly the same things as having pre-hypertension. Who could possibly know? But just to be safe, you might as well just start taking the tablets now.

In fact, a study done in Norway a few years ago looked at the issue of cholesterol and blood pressure targets in more detail. Using guidelines developed by the European Society of Cardiology (ESC) they established that, by the age of 50, over 95% of people would have a cholesterol level, or blood pressure level, considered high enough to require drug treatment.[2] This is despite the fact that the Norwegians are amongst the healthiest and longest-lived people on the planet. So God knows where that leaves the rest of us.

This same tightening of the boundaries – or some might say moving the goal posts to make more of us ill – is also happening with obesity and diabetes, where the levels considered 'normal' continue to fall. If you are an Asian Indian living in the USA or UK, you are now defined as being obese if your BMI is greater than 25. 25! That is somewhat lower than the BMI of a certain Mr Brad Pitt, and another Mr George Clooney. And, of course, chubby, chubby, me.

If we took the Norwegian figures, and added obesity, blood sugar levels, and false positives picked up on cancer screening and suchlike then I can guarantee that we would quite easily manage to make the entire population of the western world ill, in some way or another. At the same time we could ensure that we are frightened of eating, or drinking virtually anything, or doing almost anything else we enjoy.

Wherever you look, preventative medicine, and treating to ever more stringent targets, has inexorably tightened its grip on us all. Things have reached the point where I know that many people are now becoming heartily fed up with it all. Here is a copy of an e-mail that I received from a woman who had been asking for some advice about her parent's medical care. I include it, because it seems to perfectly encapsulate many people's feelings...

"I started to realise when I paid a visit to the doctor that the agenda had changed. What I wanted to discuss was increasingly irrelevant and the subject was somehow always changed to whatever it was the Department of Health had decided was 'topic of the week' – usually useless health initiatives of one sort or another.

"During the 1990s, I started receiving unsolicited demands by post that I have this test or that test. It got gradually worse and eventually whenever I visited the surgery the doctor took it on himself to bully me into letting him measure my blood pressure, have a cholesterol test, or generally badger me about 'lifestyle issues.'

"On one memorable occasion he had the cheek to ask me if 'I really had given up smoking'(!) (the answer being yes, on VJ Day 1984 – I remember the day well, not that it is anything to do with anyone else). Basically I started to feel as though I was being treated like a child who could not be trusted to make her own deci-

sions, and that this had happened gradually over the years. So I knew that something had changed and it was not I.

"I realised that the medical profession was being told what to do by the government via the Department of Health and was being encouraged to interfere in people's lives in what I regard as unacceptable ways. I started to resent the authoritarian attitude that the medical profession adopted.

"This view was compounded by the experience of seeing how my elderly mother was browbeaten by 'the experts' in the last few years of her life. Before they got their mitts on her she was relatively healthy and drug-free. By the end of her life she was a shadow of her former self – obviously some of this degeneration was only to be expected given her age. Even so..."

And all of this monitoring is going to keep on getting worse:

"The NHS future forum wants staff to routinely talk to patients about their diet to try to encourage them to eat better, reducing obesity. Patients should be asked about their diet, smoking and drinking habits every time they see a health professional according to radical proposals from the government's NHS advisers to tackle soaring rates of obesity, cancer and alcohol misuse."

Patients should be asked about their diet, smoking and drinking habits *every* time they see a health professional... Now this could become rather tiresome. One can imagine the scene in a hospital.

'Nurse, could I have a glass of water please.'

'Certainly. Now, before I give it to you, I must ask how much you smoke, how many units of alcohol you drink each day, and a breakdown of your diet in the last week.'

'Blimey, that's the tenth time I've been asked that today. Do you people not keep records of some sort?'

Perhaps that is not what the member of the NHS future forum meant when they said "*Patients should be asked about their diet, smoking and drinking habits every time they see a health professional?*" I suspect the NHS future forum has not thought things through in any great depth. They just *know* that a more intrusive and nannying approach is the way forward towards a glorious world of Überhealth.

How did we manage to reach this place?

More importantly, is this a good place to be? Has this... I am not sure exactly what to call it. Has all this monitoring, and lifelong drug taking, and obsession about healthy food and healthy behaviour made us healthier, happier and longer-lived?

No, I do not believe that it has. Or indeed ever will. Of course, some of the things we are warned about are inarguably true. Smoking causes lung cancer and heart disease, and takes about six years off your life expectancy. It also makes it far more likely that other nasty things will happen before you die – such as leg amputation and chronic lung diseases. Exercise, yes that is good for us – although putting exact figures on the benefit is more difficult, as exercise is often wrapped up with other 'healthy' behaviours.

Apart from that, what else?

The sad truth is that most of the advice we are now bombarded with varies from neutral to damaging. In some cases it can be potentially very damaging indeed. Advising people with diabetes to eat a low fat, high carbohydrate diet, for example. As a piece of harmful idiocy, this really could hardly be bettered.

How about frightening people to stay out of the sun, or slap on factor 50 cream at the first suspicion that a deadly photon may sneak through 10 layers of protective clothing. Not necessarily a good idea, because without vitamin D synthesis in the skin, from exposure to the sun, there is a significant danger that we can become vitamin D deficient, which can lead to all sorts of other problems.

Here are just two stand-out facts from a major study in the *Annals of Epidemiology* entitled 'Vitamin D for Cancer Prevention.'[3]

"Women with higher solar UVB exposure had only half the incidence of breast cancer as those with lower solar exposure."

"Men with higher residential solar exposure had only half the incidence rate of fatal prostate cancer."

To put that in simple English, if you spend longer in the sun, you may be far less likely to die of breast and prostate cancer (and lots of other cancers as well, but more on cancer later).

But what about the increased risk of dying of skin cancer! I hear you cry. Well, what of it? Around 2,000 people a year die of malignant melanoma in the UK each year. If increased sun exposure were to double this figure, we would have 2,000 more cases.

On the other hand, breast cancer kills around 20,000 a year, as does prostate cancer. If we managed to halve the rate of breast and prostate cancer, we would reduce cancer deaths by 20,000 a year. Which is ten times as great any potential increase in deaths from malignant melanoma.

(This rough calculation assumes that sun exposure actually does cause malignant melanoma – which may not be true. In fact, there is some strong evidence that sun exposure actually protects against malignant melanoma).

So we have now reached a very strange situation where people are virtually ordered to avoid the sun in order to prevent cancer. Want to find out more on this topic – that will be coming once I have managed to get a proper sun tan, and written the next book.

Have you ever heard anything of this counter evidence about sun exposure before? No, because with health advice all you ever get is one side of a story. There seems to be an utter terror that any message can contain the slightest nuance, or doubt. Sunshine is bad for you... end of discussion. Drinking alcohol is bad for you... end of discussion. Breast cancer screening is good for you... end of discussion. These absolutist positions will not admit the slightest shade of grey and believe me there are many more than 50...

And of course, this is not science. This is the world of faith and belief, or perhaps the Spanish Inquisition. A world where questioning is not welcomed, but crushed. What drives this process is, of course, fear. Fear of death and dying is hardly a new phenomenon, but it does seem to have gripped people far more strongly than at any time in history. A situation perfectly described by a very wise American doctor:

"Nothing has changed so much in the health-care system over the past twenty-five years as the public's perception of its own health. The change amounts to a loss of confidence in the human form. The general belief these days seems to be that the body is fundamentally flawed, subject to disintegration at any moment, always on the verge of mortal disease, always in need of continual monitoring and support by health-care professionals. This is a new phenomenon in our society."

Clifton Meador M.D.

If you are desperate to reassure people that all of your monitoring and screening and treating and banning is the right thing to do you will not, indeed cannot, allow people to question it.

But what if you are wrong?

What if salt is good for you, and sunshine is good for you, and being overweight is good for you, and breast screening is bad for you, and a high blood cholesterol level is good for you... what then? Then you are controlling and nannying and bullying people into doing things that are actually damaging them. In some cases, damaging them quite badly. You think that this language is too strong?

I plucked this comment from a discussion forum on breast screening:

"I'm one of the women you rarely hear from, a woman who years ago underwent invasive and disfiguring breast surgery (called a "quadrant resection") to remove a "suspicious mass" that had been identified via mammogram, but turned out to be a perfectly benign and harmless little nothing. Not only did I have to endure this deforming surgical procedure, but I also had to suffer the same extreme anxiety, fear and emotional trauma that any woman faces before going into surgery for such a reason.

"When the outcome turns out to be "Never mind! It's nothing!", relieved patients are then expected to be grateful to the brilliant surgeons who "saved" us, and the brilliant radiologists who overdiagnosed us.

"How many more of us are there out there?"

Well, how many of you are out there? Hard to say, because no one really counts women who didn't actually have cancer after all, but were still forced to endure extreme fear, and disfiguring breast cancer surgery. They may well be filed under 'success.' In fact, I know that they are.

Does this mean that breast cancer screening does more harm than good? It could mean that, but not necessarily. There are most certainly women who have early stage breast cancer picked up on screening who are 'cured'. I am also aware that many people would far rather be 'safe than sorry' at almost any cost. The idea that cancer could be missed is, for a number of women, utterly terrifying.

Which, in a slightly roundabout way takes me to the main reason why I wrote this book. It is most definitely *not* to tell people what to do. In my view there are more than enough people doing that nowadays. I am also aware that my approach to life would not be right for everyone. I am a natural risk taker, and I am therefore emotionally and philosophically uncomfortable about screening, and scanning, and monitoring and suchlike. It seems a pretty miserable way to live.

I don't know what my blood pressure is, and I don't care. I get a sun tan and even, dare I say it, get a bit sunburnt from time to time. I used to ride motorcycles, and in my reckless youth set off an avalanche when skiing off-piste, having first ducked under the avalanche warning tape.

I have friends and relatives who sit on the complete opposite end of the spectrum. One relative used to, literally, chase her children down

13

the beach, slapping factor 50 sun tan lotion onto them. She obsesses over lumps and bumps, each one a harbinger of cancer. A family friend used to clean the seats in public toilets before allowing her children to use them. For people like them, a headache is a brain tumor; a cough, lung cancer; a poke in the eye, a loss of sight. Some people like having bilateral mastectomies – just to be safe.

In short, I know that I view the world of acceptable risk from the opposite end of the spectrum to many other people. I also know that two people could be told exactly the same thing about a medical procedure, and the potential benefits and risks, yet come to completely different conclusions.

However, whatever end of the spectrum you come from, I believe it is important to know what the benefits and risks truly might be. Currently, it is almost impossible to do this. There are too many vested interests promoting only one side of the story. At the same time the information is usually presented as black or white; good or bad, with no shades of grey allowed.

Here is what Professor Michael Baum had to say on the issue of breast screening. As you may have noticed, I have focused on breast screening in this introduction as I believe it sits comfortably within the grey area between benefit and harm. There are clearly significant downsides, but it is almost always presented as an absolute good.

"After a systematic review of all websites on this subject, a recent paper in the British Medical Journal concluded that women are being coerced into screening by those organizations connected to the government or the screening industry. I am neither for nor against screening, but I am a passionate champion of informed choice for women. For an informed choice women should be treated as adults and provided with balanced information, not with propaganda."[4]

Michael Baum is not some raving nutcase. He is Professor Emeritus of surgery and visiting Professor of medical humanities at University College London. He has studied breast cancer for the best part of 30 years, and set up one of the first UK breast screening centres. This man could hardly be more 'establishment.' Yet, even he fears that women are being fed propaganda – not facts.

One form of propaganda is to ensure that the upside is presented in such a way as to make interventions seem far more impressive than they are. Here is Professor Baum again on screening for another type of cancer, prostate:

"Each year I play a game with the senior postgraduate students at a course for specialists in cancer run by the Royal College of Surgeons of England. I tell them that there are two potentially effective screening tools for prostate cancer, one which will reduce their chances of dying from the disease by between 20 and 30 per cent, while the other will save one life after 10,000 person-years of screening. As a consumer or as a public health official, which one would you buy into? They all vote for the first; yet the two programmes are the same, they were just packaged differently. To continue marketing screening in terms of relative risk reduction in breast cancer mortality is disingenuous in the extreme."[5]

Some of you may need to read that again, to understand what just happened.

- One screening tool reduces the chances of dying of prostate cancer by 20 – 30%.

- The other will save one life for every 10,000 person-years of prostate screening.

In fact they are both the same screening tool, and both results are exactly the same, just presented differently. Oh what fun you can have with statistics. Just wait until I start looking at this area in more detail. It's a laugh a minute I can promise. Pages fly by as if by magic.

But to return to breast cancer screening for a last time – in this introduction at least. The benefits are shouted from the very rooftops. Yet when it comes to the risks of over diagnosis and overtreatment... silence. On the section covering the risks of mammography, the NHS breast cancer screening website has this to say:

"Any x-ray involves radiation but mammograms only require a very low dose. It is about the same as the dose a person receives by flying from London to Australia and back. The risk that such a low dose could cause a cancer is far outweighed by the benefits of early detection of breast cancer."[6]

Oh well, bang goes my 'Have a mammogram whilst on a long-distance flight' business proposition. More seriously. That... is... it. There is nothing else on their website that talks directly about possible downsides. Nothing. A page on risk states that benefits far outweigh risks? Perhaps they should just have said that 'The only downside is that there *is* no downside.'

How can anyone possibly make their mind up when being fed propaganda such as this? The correct answer is that they cannot. You cannot. One cannot. So what information can you believe?

"If two people present diverging views on a subject, who should one trust? Which one is presenting fact and which opinion? This should be a relatively simple exercise, but because of sophistry, spin and the deliberate misinterpretation of information, it has become increasingly difficult to distinguish true facts from the plethora of dubious information with which we are bombarded... unfortunately, the misinformation explosion has swamped factual stories."

Stanley Feldman, Vincent Marks. *Panic Nation*

So you trust the experts... right?

No, I do not think that would be the best way to go. In fact, long sections of this book are dedicated to an exploration of the role of the 'expert' (chapter six). The bottom line is that experts are just as prone to grasping the wrong end of the stick as anyone else, then hanging on for blue bloody murder. Far more so, in many cases.

If truth be told, my view of medical experts has become extremely jaundiced. At times I feel they are like those highly decorated generals in North Korea with the funny hats. They look splendid, and important, but the only point of their existence is to suppress dissent and keep an idiotic regime in place. In reality, you are not likely to get much nuance from an expert. You are more likely to be 'educated' on the party line. Room 101 lurks.

So, can you rely on the information in this book? Is it perfectly balanced, and without bias? No, that would clearly be an impossible claim to make. I know that I am biased in some of my interpretations. Perhaps most importantly, as a natural risk taker I will always tend to err on the side of fewer, rather than more interventions, scanning and screening. Fewer, rather than more drugs.

If presented with the question: 'Would you prefer a shorter happy life to a longer miserable one?' I would go for short and happy every time. Although I would definitely like to know exactly how much shorter and/or happier are we talking about here? Lots of added happiness in return for very little life shortening is my goal.

In reality, you do not need to swap happiness for life expectancy. A study in 2011 called "Happiness Impacts On Lifespan Regardless Of Health Or Financial Issues", and published in the *Proceedings of the National Academies of Sciences* stated the following:

"We had expected that we might see a link between how happy people felt over the day and their future mortality, but we were struck by how strong the effect was."

If you are happy, you live longer. I suppose most people instinctively know that this is true, but nice to see it proved, and published.

However, despite my naturally risky nature, and my belief that enjoyment and happiness are good for you, I have attempted to be as balanced as I can be. My hope is that, once you have read this book, you will have far greater insight into the daily bombardment of medical scare stories and misinformation. Then, having gained this insight, you will be able to decide for yourself what to do.

I suspect that you can then happily ignore at least 95% of the healthcare advice that rains down. Coffee, good or bad? Probably neither – but it does taste good. Green leaf tea? Drink it if you want but, frankly, don't expect it to save your life in a coruscating, life-enhancing, shower of antioxidants.

The key message here is that very few things have a significant effect on health, good or bad, and most can safely be discounted as irrelevant. Some people, and most doctors, will consider this an irresponsible and dangerous approach to life. Perhaps it is. This is why I nearly called this book the Dangerous Book for Grown-Ups. Decide for yourself what you should do, take that (perceived) risk. However, the book got bigger than that, the issues rather more serious and complex.

Some years ago, I wrote a chapter in a book called *Panic Nation*, which covered many medical matters. I felt that part of the Introduction, written by Professors Stanley Feldman and Vincent Marks, summed up much of what I was trying to say.

"At the end of the day we must remember that, in the world of healthcare, things are getting better. The fact that we are living longer, healthier lives suggests that there cannot be anything terribly wrong with the air we breathe, the food we eat or the way we live.

"We must remember this, in spite of the blandishments, threats, warning and various campaigns by governments to make us eat this or that, to forgo a familiar habit or to exercise ourselves until we drop. It is a sobering thought, first expressed by John Locke in 1689 in his treatise 'A letter Concerning Toleration': 'No man can be forced to be healthful, whether he will or not?' In a free society, individuals must judge for themselves what information they choose to heed, and what they ignore."

Stanley Feldman, Vincent Marks. *Panic Nation*

10 tools for establishing the truth

How can you know what is true and what is not. Especially when it comes to information about health? Is it remotely possible to sift out what is important from meaningless noise? To know what is certain, from that which is mere speculation. To distinguish science from dogma?

The boy who cried wolf

I know that many people are so fed up with the daily bombardment that they have decided to ignore it all, basing their philosophy on the tale of "The boy who cried wolf". When they see yet another headline announcing that this substance causes cancer, or heart disease, they think. 'Yeah, yeah… and next week we will be told the exact opposite. There are only so many things that are capable of killing me, aren't there?'

To be frank, this is not a bad overall tactic. However, one day the boy will be telling the truth, the wolf really has come to eat you. You really should have listened. But how can you know when?

Here, for example, is a headline about drinking alcohol:

"Drinking 'just a little more than they should' puts people at risk of serious illness including heart disease, stroke and cancer, the government is warning. It warns regularly drinking two large glasses of wine or two strong pints of beer a day triples mouth cancer risk and doubles high blood pressure risk."[7]

BBC News Online

Boy cries wolf, or wolf coming to eat you?
Try this one:

"Health chief warns: age of safe medicines is ending. Antibiotic crisis will make routine operations impossible and a scratched knee could be fatal. The world is entering an era where injuries as common as a child's scratched knee could kill, where patients entering hospital gamble with lives and where routine operations such as hip replacements become too dangerous to carry out, the head of the World Health Organisation has warned."[8]

Front page of The Independent newspaper.

19

Boy cries wolf, or wolf coming to eat you?

Here is a headline about eating sausages, and suchlike:

"...The team from Harvard School of Public Health looked at 20 studies involving more than one million participants from 10 countries.

"On average, each 50 g serving of processed meat per day – the equivalent of a sausage or a couple of rashers of bacon – was associated with a 42% higher chance of developing coronary heart disease and a 19% higher risk of diabetes."[9]

Boy cries wolf, or wolf coming to eat you?

Personally, I enjoyed these two comments in the discussion fora, in reply to the first story about the perils of alcohol:

fishinmad

5TH FEBRUARY 2013 - 22:31
First they came for the smokers
Then they picked on the lazies
Then they came for the fatties
Now they're after the drinkers (again)
Who is next on their list?
You?

Laputa

5TH FEBRUARY 2013 - 22:44
Reply to **fishinmad**
First they came for the smokers
Then they picked on the lazies
Then they came for the fatties
Now they're after the drinkers (again)
Who is next on their list?
You?
Possibly, but I'll be fit enough to run away.

Here is another headline about cervical cancer screening, and the risk of not having a smear test:

"Women diagnosed with cervical cancer as a result of a smear test have a far better chance of being cured than women who do not go for tests, a Swedish study suggests. The researchers found a 92% cure rate after a smear test diagnosis, compared with 66% for symptoms-based diagnoses."[10]

Boy cries wolf, or wolf coming to eat you? With regard to not having a smear test, that is.

I will deal with three of these scare stories later in this book. One, I will not. That is the one we really need to be worried about, and that is antibiotic resistance. There are a couple of things you should note about this headline. One, there are no statistics, which is always a good sign that you should pay attention. Two, there are no statistics, which is always a good sign that you should pay attention.

Seeking the truth

I could go on, picking out thousands of headlines like the ones above. Go to Google, type in almost anything you can think of, alongside the words, say, cancer, or heart disease, or premature death and literally millions of hits will appear. If you want to be more scientific, go to *PubMed* (http://www.ncbi.nlm.nih.gov/pubmed/) the biomedical library website, and type in the same words. You will get much the same result with a lot more scientific jargon.

Idly wondering around *PubMed* one day I typed in the following three words "heart disease sugar" and 44,321 scientific papers appeared – in less than a second. The first paper to appear was "Association or Causation of Sugar Sweetened Beverages and Coronary Heart Disease: Recalling Sir Austin Bradford Hill."[11]

I wonder what it says. I vaguely wonder what the other 44,320 papers say, some of which will, no doubt, have absolutely nothing to do with either sugar or heart disease. Such is the way of search engines.

However, it would take about 50 years to read 44,000 full scientific papers, even if I did so non-stop. And today there will be a whole lot more because the one thing we most certainly do not do is stop contributing to the information overload. Enough, already. So, perhaps, I will just go on wondering about this issue for now. Although I do have the sense that I would rather enjoy a paper with "Recalling Sir Austin Bradford Hill" in the title.

Bradford Hill was a famous epidemiologist who worked with Richard Doll to establish, pretty much beyond any doubt, that smoking causes lung cancer. He is also renowned for recognising how difficult it can be to prove that something is a real cause of a disease, rather than merely an association. A lesson that many seem to have forgotten nowadays, where it seems that association is almost instantly taken to mean causation.

Leaving that issue aside for now, the central question remains. Is it possible to establish the importance of any given health story, and how likely is it to be – I hesitate to use the word – true. For I have found that the truth can be a very tricky little blighter to get hold of.

In fact, I try to steer clear of using the word true as much as is possible. For a fact may be correct, but virtually meaningless. For example the statement *"regularly drinking two large glasses of wine or two strong pints of beer a day triples mouth cancer risk and doubles high blood pressure risk."* I can guarantee that this is almost certainly factually correct in some tightly constrained way or another, but does it mean anything remotely important? Also, it is written in such a way as to imply causation, when causation cannot be proven.

Looking at another example, you can say that wearing bicycle helmets reduces head injuries in cycling accidents. Again true(ish). But they can also make it more likely that you will be hit by a car (because it has been shown that car drivers drive closer to you if you have a helmet on) and have a serious, rather than superficial head injury when you are hit. Or break your neck.

So, wearing a cycle helmet may be a good thing for reducing overall head injuries, once you have been hit, and if you ignore neck injuries. But, overall, bike helmets could do more harm than good. Discuss...

The reality is that, if you want to determine if something is as close to the 'truth' as possible, or to look at overall impact on health, you have to look beyond a small, well contained isolated 'fact,' or truth, and place it within the bigger picture. At which point one fact can be overturned by other, far more important, and completely contradictory fact.

For example, drinking alcohol could well increase the risk of mouth cancer three-fold. Yet, at the same time, other studies suggest that drinking alcohol could reduce the risk of dying of heart disease by up to 40%. You are around 10,000 times more likely to die of heart disease than mouth cancer. Which means that if you drink alcohol, you are far less likely to die – overall. Thus, one 'fact' is considerably more important than the other – even though they are both true.

Unfortunately, looking at the bigger picture means a hell of a lot of work. Who can really be bothered to read an entire scientific paper, then attempt to balance it against other papers in the area, then analyze all the information in a broader context? For most people life is far too short for such nonsense. Which means that we are usually left with two choices. Believe it... 'Why would anyone say this if it weren't true?' Or reject it. 'Same old rubbish.'

However, if either of these were the correct approach, I wouldn't have bothered to write this book. I do think that there is a third way, which I might call naive skepticism, if that makes any sense as a concept. Whenever I see a scary headline on some health issue I close my eyes, take a deep breath, and repeat to myself. 'It might be true, it might be true.' Rather than go for the instant: crumple, throw, bin.

Once I have forced myself to believe that something could just possibly be true I then don my natural skeptic hat... which always feels comfortable and well worn. My skepticism is driven by the knowledge that most research is far from a dispassionate search for the truth. It is usually being done for a purpose, by researchers who already have a clear end in sight.

For example, people rarely study alcohol consumption in order to find that it is good for you. They are usually doing it to prove that it is bad for you – and they will. Those who run cancer screening programs, and whose entire working life is based on finding it to be highly beneficial – will find that screening is, indeed, highly beneficial.

Vegetarians prove that eating meat is bad for us. Those who follow a 'paleo' diet, prove the exact opposite. Those who want funding for their university department will find a scare story of some sort, about something or other, which makes worldwide headlines. This will establish them firmly at the front of the queue when it comes to the next budget round.

Pharmaceutical companies spend hundreds of millions on massive clinical studies. They are determined to prove that their drug is better than any other drug, or placebo. Unsurprisingly, they mostly seem to manage this, even if the truth has to become stretched thinner than a mono layer of graphene in order to do so.

The simple fact is that you will find it very difficult to come across any research that is not biased in some way or other. Some of this is just basic human nature in action. We like to confirm, rather than confront. However, some of this bias is far from innocent. Much of it is deliberately conceived, and done with a clear end in sight.

Unfortunately, the problem of 'conscious' scientific bias has increased dramatically over the years. We have now reached the point where it has become almost impossible to understand what is being said, as facts are being manipulated for a purpose. Not always a commercial purpose, although money now plays an increasingly powerful role. This is why I used the second title for the book: *Doctoring Data*.

If you read medical papers from 50 or 60 years ago they are crystal clear, and the findings are presented in such a way that you can actually understand what the authors are trying to say. Incomprehensible statistical tests were kept to an absolute minimum. It is also difficult to spot any underlying agenda – other than an attempt to establish the truth.

Here is an extract from a paper written in 1940 about coronary heart disease – something that was becoming a major issue at the time:

"Coronary disease increases with age, and its clinical manifestations occur much less frequently in women than in men. In comparing patients with hypertension with the controls, it was therefore important that both groups show a comparable age and sex distribution. Furthermore, in studying necropsy data, one must beware of certain errors that are found in autopsy protocols. It is recognized that notes on the coronary vessels which are made during routine necropsies may not always be reliable. When the cause of death is extracardiac, the coronary vessels may not be examined with sufficient care to ascertain the extent of the atherosclerotic lesions, if any are present. If sufficient care is taken, i.e., if the three main coronary arteries are opened throughout their entire length, accurate data on the condition of these vessels can be obtained by routine dissection alone."[12]

You cannot fail to understand what is being said here. And the only agenda appears to be an attempt to understand, and explain, heart disease. However, over the years, things have become far less innocent, and I am not alone in recognising it.

The decline in honesty in science

"Anyone who has been a scientist for more than 20 years will realize that there has been a progressive decline in the honesty of communications between scientists, between scientists and their institutions, and between scientists and their institutions and the outside world.

"Yet real science must be an arena where truth is the rule; or else the activity simply stops being science and becomes something else: Zombie science. Zombie science is a science that is dead, but is artificially kept moving by a continual infusion of funding. From a distance Zombie science looks like the real thing, the surface features of a science are in place – white coats, laboratories, computer programming, PhDs, papers, conference, prizes, etc. But the Zombie is not interested in the pursuit of truth – its citations are externally-controlled and directed at non-scientific goals, and inside the Zombie everything is rotten...

"Scientists are usually too careful and clever to risk telling outright lies, but instead they push the envelope of exaggeration, selectivity and distortion as far as possible. And tolerance for this kind of untruthfulness has greatly increased over recent years. So it is now routine for scientists deliberately to 'hype' the significance of their status and performance and 'spin' the importance of their research."

Bruce Charlton: Professor of Theoretical Medicine

In a similar, if less emotive vein, the most downloaded paper in recent medical scientific literature was written by John Ionnadis. It was entitled "Why most published research findings are false."[13]

The vast majority of people have never heard of this paper. The vast majority of those who have heard of it have never read it, and the vast majority of those who have read it, have clearly not understood the implications of what they have just read. Or, if they have, they are too frightened to do anything about it.

The shortest summary of his research is, as follows:

"Moreover, for many current scientific fields, claimed research findings may often be simply accurate measures of the prevailing bias."

J. Ionnadis

These words sound relatively mild, but the implications are explosive. Basically, many researchers are claiming that they have proved something to be true, but all they have actually done is to manipulate their research in order to confirm what they already 'knew' to be true.

Does this mean they are lying? Once again we perhaps need new words here to describe human activity where the truth is not necessarily sought, or welcomed. I am certain that most researchers are convinced they are not lying, or trying to distort their findings. They would be outraged if anyone said that they were. Most scientists (if not all), do not set out to deliberately manipulate, or distort the truth.

But when the pressure is on, it is remarkably easy to dismiss a finding here, explain away a fact there, seek out studies that confirm your views, and find flaws in research that appears contradictory. Before you know it, facts can twist through one hundred and eighty degrees. Which is why two groups of researchers can look at exactly the same data, and come to completely opposed views as to their meaning. (See climate change).

If it *is* true that most research findings are just confirmation of popular bias/dogma, and personally I have no doubt that it is, how can you sift out the information that is true/accurate, and potentially vitally important, from that which is true but completely irrelevant? Or, perhaps more critically, how can you recognise the health stories which are so biased as to be – effectively – untrue. How can you find out the consequences of 'doctoring the data'?

Ionnadis, and many others, have recognised that there is a massive problem at the heart of current research, but they have not really proposed any workable solutions. Should you believe everything, or believe nothing. Trying to establish any type of system for establishing the truth is clearly not simple, and it is fraught with its own biases.

Having said this, I do think that there are certain 'tools' that you can use to analyse health stories and clinical papers. Using them will allow you to spot many of the manipulations and biases.

These tools are not complete, and they are not some sort of mathematical formula, whereby a score of five means the paper is true, and a score of ten means it is untrue. However, I believe that they can guide you, and give you a much clearer picture of what is really happening out there, in the murky world of medical research. A way of looking at the world to try and establish the truth. Or something as close to the truth as can be achieved.

The truth toolkit

Ten things to remember, to help you make sense of a medical story; they are also the chapters of this book.

- Association does not mean causation

- Lives cannot be saved; we're all going to die

- Relative mountains are made out of absolute molehills

- Things that are not true are often held to be true

- Reducing numbers does not equal reducing risk

- Challenges to the status quo are crushed – and how!

- Games are played and the players are...

- Doctors can seriously damage your health

- Never believe that something is impossible

- 'Facts' can be, and often are, plucked from thin air

CHAPTER ONE

Association does not mean causation

Of all the things you should bear in mind when looking at health stories, this is probably the single most important. Association does *not* mean causation. The reason why this is so important is that the majority of studies find only associations, yet they are presented in such a way as to imply that a cause has been found.

Here is a typical headline from the *Daily Mail*: "Eating red meat regularly 'dramatically increases the risk of death from heart disease'"[14]

It is true that this newspaper headline does not actually state that eating red meat *causes* heart disease. Not quite, but very nearly, and you could be forgiven for thinking that it does. Read it again, and you will not actually see the word 'cause'. It is just implied very strongly.

However, as you get into the article itself, any distinction between association and causation fades almost to nothing:

"Senior author Professor Frank Hu, from Harvard School of Public Health in Boston, US, said: 'This study provides clear evidence that regular consumption of red meat, especially processed meat, contributes substantially to premature death.

"On the other hand, choosing more healthful sources of protein in place of red meat can confer significant health benefits by reducing chronic disease morbidity (illness) and mortality.

"The study found that cutting red meat out of the diet led to significant benefits. Replacing one serving of red meat with an equivalent serving of fish reduced mortality risk by 7 per cent."

At this point we are heading into the territory of Bill Clinton in his impeachment trial where the meaning of words is being stretched to their very limit. At one point, after being asked a fairly direct question, he answered 'But what is, is?' (I think Wittgenstein wrote several books about this).

27

I defy anyone to read these paragraphs and not conclude the following:

1. These researchers proved that eating red meat causes premature death;

2. The researchers further proved that replacing 1 serving of red meat with fish reduced the risk of dying by 7 per cent.

I don't think you could be blamed for thinking these two things. Because that appears to be exactly what was said. Or was it? Were you just being fooled by a complex conjuring trick made up of carefully chosen words, designed to bewilder.

Here are the actual conclusions of the paper: *"Red meat consumption is associated with an increased risk of total, CVD, and cancer mortality."*

Note the word associated. Where is the word 'cause'? It is not there, because this study could not, ever, prove causality. Why not? Because it was an observational study (actually it was a review of two other observational studies). And why is this so important that makes it one of the top ten truths?

The yellow finger phenomenon

In an observational study you do not do anything active. You just carefully study the things that people do, or eat, and see if any associations emerge. If you do find an association, the next question you have to ask is the following. Are you looking at yellow fingers, or smoking?

By which I mean the following. It is clearly true that yellow fingers are associated with a higher rate of lung cancer. Does it follow that yellow fingers cause lung cancer? No, of course not. What it means is that people with yellow fingers are usually people who smoke. And smoking vastly increases the risk of dying of lung cancer.

In this case the distinction between cause of lung cancer (smoking) and an association with both (yellow fingers) is blatantly obvious – or at least it has become so after 50 years of research. Indeed, if I were now to try to claim that having yellow fingers causes lung cancer, you would look at me as though I were an idiot – and I would be. Either that, or an employee of British American Tobacco.

Yet, when a study finds that eating red meat is associated with a higher risk of heart disease, we seem to rush headlong into the conclusion that red meat consumption almost certainly does cause heart disease.

However, red meat consumption could equally just be the equivalent of yellow fingers. You think not? In that case you are probably thinking along the lines that red meat contains saturated fat, and saturated fat raises cholesterol levels, and raised cholesterol levels cause heart disease. If you immediately played this simple causal chain out in your mind, you would certainly not be alone in doing so.

Indeed, believing that we have discovered a cause (far, far, too early) is something that our brains seem hard-wired to do...

"...our brains and nervous systems constitute a belief-generating machine, an engine that produces beliefs without any particular respect for what is real or true and what is not. This belief engine selects information from the environment, shapes it, combines it with information from memory, and produces beliefs that are generally consistent with beliefs already held. This system is as capable of generating fallacious beliefs as it is of generating beliefs that are in line with truth."[15]

We cannot seem to help ourselves from linking things together to create powerful beliefs that certain things cause other things to happen. This is emotionally driven. It is an exceedingly powerful mental mechanism, and deconstructing such beliefs once they have been put together is the work of Hercules.

In this particular case, though, if you thought red meat caused heart disease by raising cholesterol levels, you must now back track and clear your mind. Because the Harvard team found that those who ate the most red meat actually had the *lowest* cholesterol levels. The table shown (figures taken from the paper itself) divides people into five groups or quintiles. Those in quintile 1 ate the least red meat, those in quintile 5 the most.[16]

Total Red Meat Intake Quintile, Servings per Day					
Quintile	1*	2	3	4	5**
% with high-Cholesterol	14.8	11.1	9.7	9.0	7.9

*(least red meat); **(most red meat)

The authors chose not to make any comment at all on this finding, although you might have thought it worth a brief mention. Had they found rising cholesterol levels with increased meat consumption you can be absolutely certain they would have presented this as a clear-cut causal chain – sometimes, though, silence shouts louder than mere words.

So, if it wasn't through raising cholesterol, how did eating red meat cause an increase in the rate of heart disease? Because it just did… through some mechanism unknown to medical science? The evil power of 'redness'.

What is far more relevant in this case is that they also found that those who ate the most red meat also smoked the most, exercised the least, ate far more calories in total, and were more likely to have diabetes. But it was the red meat that killed them from heart disease… you think?

Red meat killed them, even if, in this study, red meat included burgers, hotdogs, and other foodstuffs that no French person would consider any form of meat. And then there's the ketchup, buns and baps surrounding the 'meat.'

Leaving the weirdly manipulated details of this study aside for the moment, by far the most important point, is that this was an *observational* study only, and you *cannot* use observational studies to confirm that anything causes anything else. Studies like this merely demonstrate associations.

So quite how they then managed to say: "*The researchers further proved that cutting out red meat and replacing with fish reduced mortality risk by 7 per cent,*" is completely beyond me. Because no-one cut out anything, or replaced it with anything else. I think at this point the researchers were getting as close to a complete untruth as they could – maybe even a bit further.

The simple fact is this. If you want to know that something truly does *cause* harm, you need to do the following. You need to recruit thousands and thousands of people who are, to all intents and purposes, exactly matched. Then you have to randomly split them into two equal groups, and change one thing, and one thing only e.g. smoking, or exercise, or red meat consumption. After a few years you can find out if changing that one thing had some measurable effect; good, or bad.

This type of research would be known as a controlled, randomised, interventional study. Until you do a study like this you cannot establish causality – for certain. The simple reality is that, when you do interventional studies, the results can turn things you thought you knew completely upside down. Strongly positive associations can simply disappear. In the most extreme cases causality flips through one hundred and eighty degrees. No longer a cause, but a protective factor.

What can happen when associations are tested

One of the most powerful examples that I know of, which demonstrates how misleading observational studies can be, is from the field of Hormone

Replacement Therapy (HRT). For many years it had been recognised that younger women had far lower rates of heart disease than younger men. Younger in this case means under the age of about 50, or 60.

For various reasons it became widely accepted that younger women were protected from heart disease by their female sex hormones. Over time, this hypothesis reached the point where it had become a 'known fact.' Indeed, doctors started giving sex hormones (in the form of HRT) to menopausal women in order to continue their protection against heart disease into later life.

In 1987 a study was done which appeared to prove beyond doubt that the hypothesis was true. This study found that women taking HRT had a 42% reduction in strokes and heart disease – compared to women not taking the drugs. This seemed to be a deal clincher and so millions more women were given HRT.

So powerful did this idea become, so unquestioned, that HRT for menopausal women became incorporated into the American College of Physicians' guidelines. Failure to prescribe HRT to menopausal women was then considered medical malpractice – at least in the USA.[17]

What was somewhat overlooked in all of this is that the 1987 study was observational, not interventional, and the data were horribly biased from the start. Women who took HRT – before it became incorporated into guidelines – were a different breed. They were very health conscious, more highly educated, and from higher social groups. They smoked less, they exercised more, and they had higher paying jobs. You name a potentially confounding variable, and it varied.

Perhaps it could be argued, therefore, that this study from 1987 was not actually comparing two populations that had the same heart disease risk to start with?

Then, a few years later, something unusual happened. A controlled study was actually set up to further confirm the benefits of taking HRT. It was called the HERS study 'The **H**eart and **E**strogen/Progestin **R**eplacement **S**tudy'. Doctors stood back and waited for the expected results to arrive. Cue drum roll... da... da!

Unfortunately, the HERS study showed absolutely no impact on heart disease. And shortly after that, things got far worse. HERS was then followed by the Women's Health Initiative (WHI) study. This was the first randomised primary prevention trial to use HRT, and nearly 17,000 women were involved.

The results were, as follows:

"Analysis of hazard ratios showed that after 5.2 years, there was a 29% increase in coronary heart disease risk, including an 18% risk of coronary heart disease mortality and a 32% increase in risk of nonfatal myocardial infarction. There was a 20% increase in the risk of fatal stroke and a 50% increase in the risk of nonfatal stroke in women assigned to HRT."[18]

So a 42% *protection* in an observational study turned out to be a 29% *increased risk* in an interventional study. A complete turn-around. Findings that swept away everything that everyone thought they knew. Oops.

This should stand as a very stark warning that observational studies cannot establish anything other than associations. However powerful the associations may look, however tempting it is to believe that those associations are, indeed, causal, they can still turn out to mean nothing at all. At the extreme end, what you thought was protective is actually damaging – and *vice-versa*.

If you fool yourself into believing otherwise you will get yourself into very deep water, and can end up looking exceedingly foolish. All scientists, when you ask them, know this full well. Yet it seems that almost every day, another group of researchers will do an observational study, discover some new association, and it will be widely reported as a cause. At which point another headline will appear, such as the following:

"A soda a day raises CHD risk by 20%. Sugary drinks are associated with an increased risk of coronary heart disease (CHD)."[19]

So what does this study mean? I think we can be absolutely certain that it means nothing at all. The very paper that it was written on can be happily crumpled into a small ball and lobbed into the bin. In fact, any newspaper headline stating this or that factor raises the risk of some deadly outcome by a clearly defined 'per cent' can be ignored. This is virtually a cast-iron rule.

If the alternative is to believe that all of these associations truly are causes, then one sausage a day increases the risk of heart disease by 42%, red meat by another 20%, and a soft drink by a further 20%. Three foodstuffs and we already have an 82% increase in risk. Add in a rasher of bacon, and a pizza, and you have little chance of making it to the end of the week.

If you're off out for a takeaway already and you never pick this book up again you have just read the more important message, and you can 'take away' the message that association does not mean causation. If you do this, your life will be the richer, and simpler, for it. And probably longer as well.

CHAPTER TWO

Lives cannot be saved;
we're all going to die

Another loud warning bell should sound when a study claims to have proven that something is 'life saving', or words to that effect...

Because, sad to say, the chances of getting out of life alive are zero. Indeed, to the best of my knowledge, no-one has managed it yet. We will all die – at some point. This is one of the very few things that I know to be absolutely and completely true.

Yet, when you read the result of certain clinical studies, they will often claim that treatment x would 'save' 50,000 lives a year... if only more people were to take it. Whenever I read such things I can be heard to mutter to myself. '*So, each year, this amazing new drug creates 50,000 new immortals. They can then rise up to join the Gods on Mount Olympus, so that they may gaze down upon us, the mere mortals, who must scrape out our meager existence from the soil, before we inevitably wither and die.*'

I suppose you may think. Well, what is wrong with claiming that you can save lives? Surely this is what medicine is supposed to do. Well, yes, and if I pulled a child from a burning building, I am sure I would claim to have saved their life, whilst posing on the front page of the newspaper looking suitably modest.

However, in medical research, we have to be a little more scientific than this. When we are looking at any form of 'preventative' treatment, we need to ask a far more pertinent question. How much longer does this intervention – whatever it is – allow people to live?

When is a life saved not a life saved?

Here are three examples to try to highlight this point:

If a 6 month old girl came into my surgery with meningitis, and I injected her immediately with penicillin, and stopped her dying, or suffering any other serious effects, she could have another 80 years of perfectly healthy life ahead of her.

If a 37 year-old man were choking to death in front of me, and I used abdominal thrusts to clear the obstruction, I could have given him another 40 years of good quality life.

On the other hand, if someone drops down with a heart attack, and I defibrillate them, it is perfectly possible that they could arrest and die, half an hour later. In this case my heroic intervention would have given them a half an hour of extra life.

It is true that all of these interventions could be said to be 'life saving' in some form or another. However one form of life saving can clearly be of much greater value than the other. In the examples I have given, the added life expectancy varies from half an hour to 80 years. A difference of far greater than one million percent. Which means that you cannot use 'life saving' or 'lives saved', as a remotely useful outcome measure, as it means nothing.

In the same way, you should not use the term preventative medicine either. To *prevent* something means to stop it happening at all – ever. When it comes to death, you cannot prevent this from happening, no matter what you do, or how clever you are. The very best you can achieve is to delay the inevitable.

Of course *'delayative medicine'* does not quite have the same ring to it as preventative medicine, but that is what it should be called. I suppose if you wanted to be really clever you could call it cunctorative medicine – as cunctor is the Latin word for delay. Having said that, this is not some meaningless play on words for intellectual amusement. It has enormous implications for the treatments that are given to hundreds of millions of people worldwide.

Here is one example on the use of the term 'life saving', and the way it distorts benefit. This is the press release for the Heart Protection Study. The key bits about 'life saving' are at the beginning and the end:

"**LIFE-SAVER:** *World's largest cholesterol-lowering trial reveals massive benefits for high-risk patients.*

"*Statins are the new aspirin.*"

Professor Rory Collins

34

"Around a third of all heart attacks and strokes can be avoided in people at risk of vascular disease by using statin drugs to lower blood cholesterol levels – irrespective of the person's age or sex, and even if their cholesterol levels do not seem high. That's the conclusion of UK researchers who have just completed the world's largest randomised trial on cholesterol-lowering therapy.

*"Unveiling the key findings today (Tuesday 13 November) at the American Heart Association's Scientific Sessions 2001, lead researcher Professor Rory Collins said: 'This is a stunning result, with massive public health implications. We've found that cholesterol-lowering treatment can protect a far wider range of people than was previously thought, and that it can **prevent** strokes as well as heart attacks.*

*"In this trial, 10 thousand people were on a statin. If now, an extra 10 million high-risk people worldwide go onto statin treatment, **this would save about 50,000 lives each year** – that's a thousand a week."*[20]

You can review the entire press release on-line if you wish. The important things to note here are the two key concepts used, namely: 'prevention' and 'life saving'. It all sounds highly impressive and, of course, it is meant to. No-one has ever accused those involved in researching statins of hiding their light under a bushel. (Only the money they get paid).

The first problem with this press release, amongst so many others, is that no-one's life can possibly have been saved. Everyone in this study was going to die – in fact very few of those recruited are now still alive. It was certainly true that, at the end of the study, more people taking the statin were alive than those taking the placebo. But the key question 'how much longer would they live, or did they live?' was neither asked, nor answered.

If anyone had thought to ask this, what would the answer be? Would it be 80 years? Not very likely, as the average age of the participants was close to 60 – and everyone in the study was at very high risk of dying of heart disease. You only got enrolled in this study if you already had: diagnosed heart disease; diabetes; a previous stroke; or all three.

Was it ten years?

Was it a year?

No. It was around three months.

If I had been writing this press release, I might have re-worded it slightly. Bear with me here, whilst I add in another important point. As you may have noted, you would need to treat ten million people to end up with fifty thousand more alive after a year. In reality, the true figure is much closer to forty than fifty thousand, but what's an error of ten thousand deaths between friends?

It is also quite clear that the gigantic and faintly ridiculous denominator of ten million was chosen so that you could generate a headline claim of a thousand lives a week *saved*. If, however, you want to get a clearer handle on what this study actually found, it is best to reduce the numbers to a more manageable size. The simplest way to do this is to divide the ten million by fifty thousand. This leaves you with two hundred.

So, what this study really demonstrated is that you need to treat *two hundred* people for one year, for *one* extra person to be alive – at the end of that year. (This is exactly the same ratio as ten million to fifty thousand btw).

At this point it would be possible to create an even more negative (though accurate) spin to state that, if you treat 200 people, 199 of them will gain absolutely no benefit at all. The one lucky person that does benefit is likely to live for a few more months before they, too, inevitably, die.

Bearing this in mind, here is my press release:

'This trial demonstrates that if you treat two hundred people with a statin for one year, one hundred and ninety nine will die on exactly the same date as they would have done anyway. The one person in two hundred who does benefit will live for a few extra months.'

Which is a different way of saying exactly the same thing as the researchers said. But I suspect that it doesn't fill you with the same warm and positive glow. You might even feel a twinge of disappointment.

Ah yes, the power of words, and how to use them. The power of the concept of life saving, or lives saved. Such power that it has resulted in over six million people in the UK taking a statin each and every day, for the rest of their lives. At a cost of well over two billion pounds a year to the UK economy, when you take all costs into account. With another six million people shortly to start.

But to return to the main point here. Most of us take a 'preventative' drug in order to live longer. Yet, we are *never* told how much longer we are likely to live. If you think not, then here is a test for you. If you are on a statin, or your GP is haranguing you to take one, ask them how much longer you are likely to live if you take it? i.e. What is the average increase in survival time?

I can guarantee here and now that they will not be able to answer this question. They will either say that they do not know, or just guess, and they will guess something like five to ten years. I know this because

I have asked many doctors and nurses this exact same question. Some say ten years, some a couple of years. No-one gets anywhere near the vanishingly small figure.

Strange, is it not, that the most important fact about the benefit of statins is missing. I call this the dog that did not bark. The statin of the Baskerville's.

How cancer gets it right

One of the other things that I find fascinating about this whole area is that cancer researchers have always clearly acknowledged that you cannot save lives – or at least that is not your primary goal. The main outcome measure in cancer treatment has always been 'increase in median survival. Here is an example:

"At the American Society of Clinical Oncology Conference in June 2010, the Bristol-Myers Squibb pharmaceutical company reported the clinical findings of their drug ipilimumab. The study found an increase in median survival from 6.4 to 10 months in patients with advanced melanomas treated with the monoclonal ipilimumab, versus an experimental vaccine."[21]

So if you take ipilimumab (if you can pronounce it) for about ten months then you will live, on average, 3.6 months longer than if you do not. Sorry, but even that sentence is not entirely accurate as median and average survival are not the same thing. They can be, but usually they are not.

Ignoring this issue for now, and using average rather than median, I put it to you, the members of the jury, that a 3.6 month increase in survival is not very impressive. Or is it? I don't really know. If those extra 3.6 months were spent in agony from some horrible side-effect – most certainly not.

If they were spent with a supportive and loving family around – most certainly so. Unless you are a health economist, who would no doubt sit by the side of your bed with a clipboard, tapping their pen, and shaking their heads at the waste of taxpayers' money. *'I hope you realise you are costing the NHS £200,000 a year...'*

However, the main point I want to make here is that, in the world of cancer, the concept of increased life expectancy is almost universally used, and widely accepted, and that is pretty much that. Yet, in the world of heart disease, you will never hear anyone mention this outcome. Why are they so different?

Well there are a number of interconnected reasons for this, but I shall try to keep it very simple. Historically, once you got cancer, you were unlikely to be cured. It was expected that you were going to die of the disease. So the primary concern was – how long does the patient have left to live? The net result of asking this question is that most people involved in cancer treatment started off by trying to increase survival time, not necessarily achieve a 'cure'. Although 'cures' are, in fact, now possible.

Effectively, the world of cancer treatment grew from a rather more humble place, where doctors and researchers were just trying to give people more time on the planet. Cardiologists, on the other hand, were curing, and preventing, and saving lives left, right, and centre. *'Have at thee, heart disease!'* Ah, what a bold and exciting place to be.

How powers that be value a life

However, the net result of this, is that it has made cardiology interventions appear far, far, more impressive than they really are. And oncology (cancer) treatments, appear far, far, worse. To return to ipilimumab for a moment:

*"The National Institute for Clinical Excellence (NICE) has recommended in a draft guidance **against** Bristol-Myers Squibb's Yervoy (ipilimumab) for the treatment of advanced malignant melanoma in patients who have already been treated with chemotherapy. NICE decides whether a drug, medical device or treatment should be covered by the National Health Service (NHS), the country's universal health care service."[22]*

As I had rather expected, NICE turned ipilimumab down, on the basis that it costs far too much for the rather puny clinical benefit – plus, no-one had a chance of spelling it correctly. But is the benefit really that puny? Treatment for under a year means an average increase of life expectancy of three point six months – and that is (on average) **for every single person taking the drug**.

Compare and contrast with statins, these miracle life-savers, saviours of humanity. If you use them in the highest heart disease risk group possible, and you 'treat' for a year, the average increase in life-expectancy is around three months. However, that three months is only available for 1 person in 200. The other 199 get no added life expectancy at all.

In short, statins are very nearly 200 times *less* effective at increasing life expectancy – over one year of treatment – than ipilimumab. A drug which was *turned down* by NICE due to its lack of efficacy. But of course, statins *'save lives'*, whilst ipilimumab only allows people to live longer. It's a no-brainer. Heroism vs. pragmatism.

To be completely accurate, NICE turned down ipilimumab because they considered that it was not cost-effective. The measurement used by NICE to establish cost-effectiveness is the cost per Quality Adjusted Life Year (QALY).

One Quality Adjusted Life Year is assumed to be one extra year of perfect quality life, or two years of fifty per cent quality life, or four years of twenty five per cent quality etc. Quite how well quality of life can be measured is a complex question, and is up for much debate – most of which debate never occurs, because it is too hard, and our brains hurt.

Moving back to cost-effectiveness. It has been decreed by NICE that one QALY should cost the NHS no more than around £20,000 or £30,000. Any more than this and the intervention will be deemed too expensive.

Sorry about the vagueness of this cost per QALY number. But trying to pin NICE down to an exact figure is, frankly, impossible. This ever-moving range of £20-30,000 was simply plucked out of thin air anyway. If you think not, try to find out where it came from – and good luck with that.

So, whilst a NICE appraisal is usually a document of some several hundred pages, the basic equation at the heart of it remains the same. If each added QALY costs more than £30,000 then NICE will turn down the medical intervention. Unless, of course, it is too politically sensitive so do to – which is quite often.

On this basis ipilimumab was bound to fail. A complete course of ipilimumab consists of four injections at twenty thousand pounds a pop. Which is a total of £80,000. It extends life by around 3.6 months. Therefore, the cost per QALY (assuming those 3.6 months consisted of 100% perfect health) is £266,666. Bong, reject.

Why it takes NICE about a year to do these assessments is beyond me. Two minutes is about all you realistically need to answer three basic questions:

- How much does the intervention cost?

- What is the extension in life?

- What is the quality of life during the above extension of life?

But I suppose that if you are turning down cancer drugs then you are obliged to give the impression you have spent months thinking about all the issues in detail to the point where your brain bleeds. Also, that you have consulted all the stakeholders... God, I hate that word.

Anyway, what of statins in comparison. Admittedly the drug costs of statins are far, far, lower than ipilimumab. A patient taking a statin for a year would cost the NHS around £100, absolute minimum – if you include blood tests, GP appointments etc Which is some eight hundred times less than a course of ipilimumab.

Assuming this cost is correct – and I am deliberately underestimating costs with statins – we can do a simple thought experiment.

Statins are 199 times less effective at extending life than ipilimumab. However, they are 800 times cheaper. Which means that, the cost per QALY for statins turns out to be four times less. Which is around £66,000 per QALY.

As you may have just noticed, this is far more than the NICE cost per QALY threshold. Why, then, does NICE consider statins to be highly cost-effective? Because they don't look at the same outcome measures for cardiovascular drugs as they do with cancer drugs. Which is more than a little unfair on cancer patients, I feel.

In cardiovascular trials NICE will look at the number of extra people alive at the end of the study, and consider this to be the number of 'lives saved' by the treatment. Or the number of deaths 'prevented'. But lives saved, and deaths prevented, as discussed earlier, are completely meaningless outcome measures. A life saved represents a life extension that could range from 1 hour to 80 years.

As far as our 'truths' are concerned, the take away message from all of this is straightforward. When you see the words 'lives saved', or any version thereof, you must repeat this little mantra. 'You cannot save a life, all you can do is delay death.' You will also know that anyone who combines the words 'saved' and 'life', or any version thereof, with regard to a clinical trial, is no longer a scientist. They have effectively – if unconsciously – become a drug salesperson. However academic they may claim to be.

CHAPTER THREE

Relative mountains are made out of absolute molehills

Risk is one of the most difficult concepts to explain, or understand. Our understanding of risk is also underpinned by emotions, rather than rational thinking. This is well known by researchers, pharmaceutical companies, governments and, of course, advertising agencies.

People are often terrified of things that are extremely unlikely to happen. For instance, their child being abducted by a stranger, or a shark attack, or their child dying of meningitis. On the other hand, we happily drive cars, and smile at hippopotamuses thinking them charming and clumsy. Many people also smoke cigarettes and manage to suppress the current and future impact it will have on their health.

We fear what frightens us, and that is not necessarily what kills us.

The reality is that car crashes kill over 1,000,000 people each year worldwide, or 3,500 every day. In the UK it is about 8 a day. Deaths that we never hear of, unless they are particularly gruesome or unfortunately someone that we know. Hippos kill more humans than sharks, and alligators, and crocodiles and lions and tigers combined. I don't know what the ratio of smoking-related deaths to meningitis deaths might be. A million-to-one?

And what animal should we really, really, fear. Why, the mosquito, of course. Mosquito bites kill far more people than the bites of any other animal by a factor of several thousand. However, it would be a bit inconvenient to run screaming in terror from every mosquito you saw.

Another problem with our perception of risk is that, when we fear something, we tend to vastly overestimate the likelihood that it will happen. A study in the US in 1995 found that women overestimated their probability of dying from breast cancer within the next 10 years by a factor of 20.[23]

At the same time, fear also leads us to overestimate the protection we can gain from taking affirmative action. In the same study where women wildly *overestimated* their risk of developing breast cancer it was found that they also *overestimated* the potential benefits to be gained from breast cancer screening by a factor of 100. Taking these figures together, women are getting the risk-benefit equation wrong in breast screening by a factor of 2,000 – just for starters.

None of this is helped by the fact that the true risk of something happening is often hidden behind horribly misleading statistics. Frequently, these statistics are used in such a way that it is virtually impossible to understand the impact of what is being said.

Absolute vs. relative risk

One of the most popular forms of obfuscation is to use the term 'relative risk reduction' (RRR). Or just risk reduction (RR). I don't know when this first started, but I think that it should definitely stop. Here, for example, is a section from a patient information website on high blood pressure.

"...it is estimated that reducing a high diastolic blood pressure [the lower number] by 6 mmHg reduces your relative risk of having a stroke in the future by about 35-40%, and reduces your relative risk of developing heart disease by about 20-25%. Larger reductions in blood pressure provide greater benefits."

This all sounds very impressive. A risk reduction of 35-40%. That is nearly a half... isn't it? In truth, this small snippet of information is more honest than most. In that it does clearly state that these figures represent a *relative* risk reduction. Most information would just say... reduces risk by 35-40% with no mention of the fact that this is actually a relative risk.

Having said this, their use of the word 'relative' is still going to be pretty meaningless to most people. A risk is a risk, isn't it? Well no, not at all. Some years ago I asked 50 doctors what was the difference between 'relative' and 'absolute' risk. One doctor knew – he was deputy chief medical officer for Scotland at the time – so I guess it was probably part of his job description.

If the vast majority of doctors don't really know the difference between absolute and relative risk, what chance is there that most patients would understand this concept... virtually none.

So, I hear you cry, what does relative risk mean, and why is it different to absolute risk – and why should I care? Someone once told me the difference between absolute and relative risk is the difference between addition and multiplication. I think it is a little more complicated than this, but here goes with an example.

One hundred people start taking a blood pressure medication and one hundred do not. At the end of a year, one person in the group taking the medication has died; and two people in the group not taking medication have died.

- The absolute difference in deaths is 1 person per 100 vs. 2 people per 100 = 1 in 100, or 1%.

- The relative difference in deaths is 1 vs. 2 (½ = 50%).

I shall now claim that if you take my medication, your risk of dying has been reduced by 50% i.e. halved (which is true – sort of).

Let's try this again, with numbers that are 10 times as big.

1,000 people start taking a blood pressure medication and 1,000 do not. At the end of a year, 1 person taking medication has died, and 2 people not taking the medication have died.

- The absolute difference in deaths is 1 person per 1,000 or 0.1%.

- The relative difference is 1 vs. 2 (½ = 50%).

I shall now also claim that if you take my medication, your risk of dying has been reduced by 50% (which is also true – sort of).

But, but, but. Yes, but, but, indeed. In the first scenario, the absolute benefit was 10 times greater than in the other. However, the relative risk reduction remains *exactly* the same. Given this, what does relative risk reduction actually mean? It means, my friend, almost nothing at all. It is most often used as a technique to inflate the benefit of taking drugs.

Of course risk(s) can also be used the other way round. To scare you away from doing something the medical profession does not approve of, such as drinking. Which is a bit ironic, since most doctors are all virtually alcoholic – or maybe that's just me.

At this point, let me take you back a few pages to the short press release on the terrors of drinking alcohol... "*...regularly drinking two large glasses of wine or two strong pints of beer a day triples mouth cancer risk and doubles high blood pressure risk.*"

Triples mouth cancer risk! Yes, by golly, this statement has a sort of a truth contained in it in a relative risk sort of way, and an association not causation sort of way. But before we all run screaming in terror from the nearest Budweiser (apart from the fact that it tastes of nothing at all), we need to know the following. What is the absolute risk of dying of mouth cancer in the first place? For the UK, at least, the answer is around: 2.5/100,000[24].

That is, for every 100,000 people in the UK who die, 2.5 will do so from mouth/oral cancer. The other 99,997.5 will die of other things instead. I feel sorry for the point five. Or to put this another way. Your risk of dying of mouth cancer in the UK, at the present time, is 0.0025%. Does that seem high, or low, to you? I know it seems pretty low to me.

Now, if you were to triple that risk, it becomes 0.0075%. Is that a risk that you are willing to take? Of course, this is your choice, I am just giving you the absolute figures, without throwing in relative risk to confuse things.

I would add that this risk of 0.0025% includes smokers. If you do not smoke, your risk of dying of oral cancer is two thirds less. It is 0.00075%. Therefore, tripling it brings it back up to 0.0025% again. I apologise for all these zeros, but when you are dealing with risks this small, a lot of zeros to the right of the decimal point are the name of the game.

At this point I feel I should mention another 'association' problem here. Which is that people who drink are also more likely to smoke, less likely to take exercise, and also have other very unhealthy lifestyle factors. Any of which could be the cause of increased risk of mouth cancer. In short, this reported tripling of risk with alcohol consumption may not even be caused by the drinking at all. It may just be an association.

Anyway, assuming it is true that drinking a moderate amount of alcohol increases the risk of fatal mouth cancer, if you drink (some never quantified amount) you will increase your absolute risk of dying of mouth cancer by 0.0048% If, on the other hand, you are a non-smoker, your risk is increased by 0.0016%. A tripling of risk from bugger all, to precisely three times bugger all.

Moving on. As for drinking being alleged to double the risk of developing high blood pressure. What does this mean? To be honest, I cannot really work this out at all. As mentioned earlier, the risk of developing high blood pressure at some point in your life is already believed to be at least 90%... allegedly. How can a 90% risk be doubled? 180% does seem a bit of an extreme figure. An 80% greater risk than 100%?

I suppose you could reverse this, and say that 10% of people are not going to develop high blood pressure, and if you did not drink, that figure would increase to 20%? A doubling of a decrease in risk? And how do they know – how can they be so certain?

However, even if you did this strange thing, there is another problem to throw into this confused melting pot. Which is that the definition of high blood pressure continues to fall, and will inevitably continue to fall further in the future. So what is the definition of high blood used here – is high really high? So presumably the risk of having high blood pressure will increase from 90%. What happens when it reaches 95%, or 100% – which it will, inevitably, do? How then will they explain the people who don't get high blood pressure?

Things get even more complex if you decide to delve deeper and ask, well, how much does drinking alcohol raise the blood pressure anyway? If it is only a little bit, the risk of anything happening because of this would be increased only a little bit, as per mouth cancer.

The fact is that, the more you look into this statement, the more the questions mount up. In order to make sense of it, you need to know:

- What is the absolute increase in risk of developing high blood pressure – non drinker vs. drinker? And what is the definition of high blood pressure?

- What is the actual increase in blood pressure?

- What is the added risk of this increase in blood pressure in developing cardiovascular disease (absolute risk, not relative)?

- What is the added risk, absolute, that this increased risk of cardiovascular disease will reduce your life expectancy – and by how much?

As I hope is now clear, you can make a statement that drinking alcohol doubles the risk of developing high blood pressure, and it will probably hold true in some extremely restricted way or another. You have to ask yourself: but what does it actually mean? And how likely is this to cause significant harm?

Even if drinking alcohol does raise blood pressure, you should bear something else in mind at this point. Analysis of death rates shows that people who drink a moderate amount generally live longer than people who do not drink at all. Mainly because of a reduction in heart disease and stroke which – you guess it – are supposed to be caused by having a raised blood pressure. More on this later.

Anyway, to return to the main topic here which is the use, or misuse, of relative risk. The term is not completely useless, but it is increasingly used to inflate extremely small risks, or exaggerate marginal benefits. As such it is almost deliberately confusing and as a general rule relative risk should be ignored.

My advice is to look for absolute risk every time. If the absolute risk is hidden away, then you can confidently assume that it is so vanishingly small that the authors chose not to highlight it, as it would significantly weaken their message.

Number Needed to Treat

To be honest, I am not the only person to have recognised the range of problems encountered with using relative risk. Some years ago, a moderately successful attempt was made to introduce a different outcome measure into medical literature. It was called the Number Needed to Treat (NNT). This is more closely related to the absolute risk so it is a little better, but what does it mean?

If I can take you back to my blood-pressure lowering example from a couple of pages ago – where 100 people were given meds and 100 people weren't and then 1,000 etc. In the first case, you would need to treat one hundred people for one year to prevent one death. So the NNT = 100. In the second case you need to treat one thousand people for one year to prevent one death NNT = 1,000.

By using the NNT, it becomes quickly apparent that the one form of treatment is ten times as effective as the other. Which means that NNTs have one major advantage over using relative risk reduction, in that they come closer to establishing the absolute benefit.

However, if you have been paying attention, you will have noticed my deliberate mistake with NNTs. Which was to include the word 'prevent'. Because, and here I am at a distinct risk of repeating myself into a state of insensible coma, you cannot prevent death. You can only delay it.

Therefore, as with relative risks, benefits can still be vastly overestimated with NNTs. At least they are when you are in the world of preventative medicine. Whilst it is clearly important to know if one more person is alive at the end of a study, it is considerably *less* important if he, or she, dropped dead half an hour after the study ended.

NNTs cannot tell you this, yet NNTs are what NICE use to calculate cost per QALY. However much they may try to argue that it is far cleverer than this, it isn't.

NNTs have other problems too. Such as defining the treatment time. An NNT where you need to treat for one week to achieve a clinical benefit is clearly far better than one where you need treat for twenty years. Mostly, NNTs don't include this 'length of time' figure. Obviously they can, but quite often the authors choose not to mention it – I wonder why.

Having just said this, somewhat counter-intuitively, NNTs can be made to look better by increasing the length of time you 'treat' for. If you treat blood pressure for a year to 'prevent' one death per one hundred people, the NNT is 100. You can then treat for two years to 'prevent' two deaths, at which point the NNT is 50. If you treat for five years to 'prevent' five deaths the NNT is 20. Same drug, same effect, yet the NNT can be adjusted to make treatment appear five times more effective. A simple, yet effective, trick when you do not wish to compare like with like.

Possibly the greatest weakness of NNTs is that you are allowed to jam various end-points together to make NNTs look better. Don't just look at death. Add death to hospitalisation, non-fatal stroke, and revascularization (this is an old statin trick), and you can create the wonderful 'combined end-point NNT'. By doing this you can squeeze an NNT of 200 down to about 3, or less. Wot fun.

Yes, it is almost magical how far statistics can be manipulated, and still remain 'true,' or not a lie, or whatever form of words you feel most comfortable with.

Pharmaceutical companies long ago worked out how to make your NNTs look as bright and shiny as possible. They regularly use the 'extended treatment time' and 'combined end-point' techniques with ruthless efficiency. These two tricks can make treatments look hundreds of times better than they actually are.

Without going into this area in any more detail, it is true that NNTs are a better outcome measurement than relative risk, but they remain significantly flawed (and the moment they appeared, various agencies immediately started twisting and mangling them to produce figures to suit their argument). So, it is true that NNTs can tell you how many people you need to treat to 'prevent' something unpleasant from happening... But:

- They do not tell you how long you need to treat for (usually);

- They do not tell you how long it takes for the thing you 'prevented' from happening in the end to happen;

- You can combine NNTs from various end-points together to create a horribly misleading picture of the benefits of a treatment.

If a relative of yours is refused a new cancer drug, you can probably blame NNTs. There are other major problems with NNTs as well, but that will do for now.

Overall mortality

And now we come to another major can of worms. Eventually, as you know by now, you cannot reduce overall mortality, as we are all going to die. However, the concept of overall mortality, as reported in clinical trials, remains important enough to require further explanation. Primarily to discuss the different ways that it is used to report the results of medical studies. Or, once again, *mis*report the results of medical studies.

In many studies, the most important end-point is the number of people alive, or dead, at the end of it. If you restrict yourself to looking at one form of death e.g. cancer mortality, you can virtually do what you like with the other figures, and promote a whole series of utterly ridiculous conclusions.

For example, I could carry out a study on the effect of pushing people off high cliffs onto rocks to establish the effect on cancer mortality. As is immediately obvious, every single person I pushed off the cliff would die a few seconds later, if the cliff were high enough! However, none of them would die of cancer. Which means that I could, if I so wished, entitle my study: *'Benefits of pushing patients off a cliff on overall cancer mortality.'* **Abstract:** We have found that when patients with cancer are pushed off a high cliff this reduces mortality from cancer deaths by 100%. This represents an unprecedented reduction in cancer mortality, and we suggest this technique might be used to reduce cancer deaths around the world.

I would follow this with my seminal study on *'Removing the human brain to prevent strokes.'*

Yes, there is an obvious flaw in both of these studies. Well, more than one flaw, but the point remains. If you decide to look at only one form of mortality e.g. cancer, or stroke deaths, you can make completely idiotic claims about the benefits of your form of treatment on specific forms of mortality.

You can also make equally idiotic claims about the harm of various activities. For example, drinking alcohol – for some reason I seem to use alcohol consumption a lot. Anyway, here is a quote from an article in the *Daily Telegraph*, where researchers were claiming that the guidelines for alcohol consumption have been set far too high:

"... scientists published research recommending that 'people should cut their consumption to just 50ml of wine a day, or a quarter of a pint of beer'. If they did so... 'There would be 2,600 fewer deaths from cancer and almost 3,000 less (sic) from liver cirrhosis', they found."[25]

A... quarter... of... a... pint... of... beer... a... day... Exactly what planet do these numpties live on? There would be surely no end to the joy of daily life if the 'experts' ever managed to grab the levers of power.

As with all such studies, the figures sound initially impressive. 2,600 fewer deaths from cancer, and almost 3,000 fewer from liver cirrhosis may sound like a lot. Why that's... let me see... socks off... by golly, that's 5,600.

However, the UK has a population of around 65,000,000. So, although this sounds like a lot of deaths, 5,600 represents an extremely small percentage of the population. Also note that there is no explanation of the 5,600 figure. Is this 5,600 per day, per year, or the total number of deaths within the entire population that is alive today (which would be 1/11,600).

Back to the main theme. What we are looking at here is overall mortality, so we need to move beyond specific causes of death, to all causes of death. The best way to do this, in the area of alcohol consumption, is to type the words 'moderate alcohol consumption 'and' overall mortality,' into *PubMed*. This brings up a whole series of studies which find that moderate alcohol consumption actually reduces overall mortality... which means that, yes, you live longer.

Here is just one such paper, from the USA:

"Estimated all-cause mortality HRs (Hazard Ratios)[ii] for moderate drinkers were generally somewhat lower when compared with infrequent drinkers [Hazard Ratio for male moderate drinkers = 0.87, 95% confidence interval (CI)[iii] = 0.75-1.01 and HR for female occasional moderate drinkers = 0.80, 95% CI = 0.69-0.93]."[26]

---

ii A Hazard Ratio (HR) of 1.0 = average risk. HR 1.2 = 20% increase in risk.
iii A Confidence Interval (CI) of 95% captures the range into which 95% of results fall. If the CI includes 1.0, this is described as not statistically significant.

Here we have hazard ratios, confidence intervals etc. Stripping out the jargon what we discover is that, in moderate drinkers there is a 13% (relative risk) reduction in overall mortality, for men, and 20% relative risk reduction for women. In this case moderate drinking was taken to mean two drinks a day.

The simple fact is that if you choose to look beyond individual mortality rates it becomes very clear that moderate drinking actually reduces overall mortality. Unfortunately, I cannot tell you what moderate drinking might be, as the definition of moderate drinking is never the same in any paper I have read... ever. It ranges from around one to four units a day... sometime more, occasionally less.

However, the take away message here is straightforward. When it comes to moderate alcohol consumption you can add together deaths from mouth cancer, liver disease, increases in breast cancer, and all the other diseases that have been associated with drinking alcohol and IGNORE them.

Yes, deaths from these conditions are increased if you drink alcohol. However, the overall mortality rate is lower, so alcohol (or the lifestyle associated with drinking alcohol) is reducing the death rate from other disease by a greater amount. Add everything together and what do you get? A longer, and probably a happier, life if you drink moderately.

Of course, there has to come a point where the quantity of alcohol you drink causes enough harm that it will decrease your life expectancy. But where, exactly, is that point? No-one knows. In fact, no-one has the faintest idea. However, that is not really the point that I am trying to make here.

The point I want to make here is that, despite the limitation that we all eventually die, you must *always* look for overall mortality – wherever possible. Dying of specific diseases is, of course, important. But when people start quoting specific mortality rates, your 'Doctoring Data' antennae should start twitching madly.

Those who quote specific death rates, and keep silent about overall mortality are usually trying to hide something. Usually the effect on overall mortality, which will be unchanged, or heading off in the opposite direction to the one they want.

Here, for example, is a set of graphs created from the West of Scotland Coronary Prevention Study (WOSCOPS).[27]

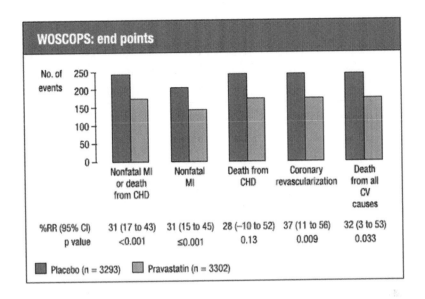

The text states that:

"This landmark study showed for the first time that statin treatment of hyper-cholesterlaemic patients without CHD not only lowers LDL but reduces fatal and non-fatal CHD events rates."

All of this is true, and we have five graphs demonstrating impressive reductions in different forms of mortality. But what was the impact on overall mortality? Well, it was not mentioned, so you are allowed to have a wild guess. Yes, you're right, it was unchanged.

On the other hand, here are the results from the 4S study (Scandinavian Simvastatin Survival Study).

*"The 4S is also the first clinical trial to clearly demonstrate that cholesterol-lowering therapy reduces the risk of **all-cause mortality** and major coronary events in CHD patients ≥65 years of age. Simvastatin treatment produced a highly significant 34% reduction in risk for all-cause mortality (P=.009), attributable to a 43% reduction in risk for CHD mortality (P=.003)."[28]*

This is just to make it crystal clear that, when there are benefits on overall mortality, this will be, almost without exception, the first outcome that is trumpeted.

Although it is slightly tangential, I feel the need to highlight something extremely important that has been left out about the 4S study. Something which you will never read, or hear spoken of... ever. Which is that, in the 4S study, more women taking simvastatin died than women taking the placebo. Admittedly there were not that many women in this study, but it is an interesting fact... no?

Overall mortality was also unchanged in women in the Heart Protection Study (HPS). Once again this fact could not be found anywhere in the original study nor, indeed, anywhere else. Until, that is, a follow up paper was published on-line five years later – with no accompanying press release. Only a deafening silence could be heard.

In fact, in no statin study done has there been an impact on overall mortality in women. None, ever. Despite this we are told, in all seriousness, that statins work just as well for women, as men. Ho, ho. (I reserve my doctoring data joker card to exclude one study from this comment. The JUPITER study, for reasons that will become obvious later).

That was a slight divergence into my area of maximum obsession. My main theme in this section is to make it clear that when you are looking at the results of a clinical study, or reading a newspaper article, you must strain your ears to listen for the dog that did not bark. Otherwise known as overall mortality. If this information is not right up there at the front, in bold, then you can be confident that it did *not* change. Crumple, throw, bin. Once again – your waste paper basket should be getting quite full by now!

You only die once

There is another issue to do with overall mortality that I also need to bring up at this point. It is the principle that *'You can only die once, of one thing.'*

This basic principle may seem pretty simple, but it appears to have passed by almost all researchers, especially in heart disease research. For example, in the sixties, seventies and eighties... a time before statins. Yes, there was a time before statins. It was stated that drugs which lowered cholesterol levels also reduced deaths from heart disease.

However, they did *not* affect overall mortality. In many cases overall mortality increased. By which I mean that more people in the cholesterol lowering 'intervention' arm were dead at the end of the study.

Against all principles of logic, this evidence has been used to promote the idea that cholesterol lowering did actually reduce death from heart disease. It is argued that, yes, yes, the overall mortality rate did go up. However, the rate of deaths from heart disease went down. Which was taken as proof that lowering cholesterol prevented heart disease, prior to the introduction of statins.

Or, to put this another way, cholesterol lowering is clearly a good thing, but other adverse effects of these drugs must have overcome the cholesterol lowering benefits in reducing heart disease. Further proof that the cholesterol hypothesis must be true.

Hmmmm. Good try, but completely idiotic.

The reality is this. If more people die from other causes, then there are fewer people left to die of heart disease. As with throwing people off cliffs to prevent deaths from cancer. If you give people a drug that increases deaths from cancer you cannot then die of heart disease.

The reason why the rate of deaths from heart disease went down in the pre-statin cholesterol lowering trials is precisely *because* the rate of death from other causes went up. This is simple logic. Page one, sentence one.

This was explained to me in another way by a fellow doctor who often states that: 'Cholesterol lowering may change what is written on your death certificate, but it won't change the date.'

The final game played with overall mortality is to dismiss it, when it has not been altered, as being irrelevant. This will be done by claiming that no difference could be seen because the clinical study was 'not powered' to show any difference in this outcome.

I hope it is now becoming clear that there is almost no end to the way that data are doctored Almost everywhere you look there are scientists and researchers playing exceedingly clever games with the data in order to promote their favoured message.

I certainly have sympathy with any Government trying to create laws to prevent tax avoidance. Five minutes after you publish your exceedingly complex guidelines, 10,000 tax lawyers have worked out 8,000,000 different ways of getting round them.

·In medical research there are hundreds of different ways of choosing how to present the data to make them seem to say certain things. None of these are direct lying (tax evasion), they are just ways of twisting meaning through virtually 180 degrees (tax avoidance).

Where was I? Oh yes, the trick of dismissing a lack of change in overall mortality as unimportant, because the trial could not have shown it – statistically speaking.

The null hypothesis

This technique starts at the very beginning of a clinical trial whereby, before you start, you try to work out how many people you need to recruit to show a statistically significant change in an outcome e.g. death. The technical phrase for this process is 'disproving the null hypothesis.' The null hypothesis is that the two things you are measuring are the same. Disproving it means that they are not.

If you treat two groups of people with a drug vs. placebo, the null hypothesis is that you will not see any significant difference. If you do, you have disproven the null hypothesis, and you can state that your drug did have a significant effect – hopefully beneficial.

The bigger the difference you expect to see, the fewer people you need to recruit into your trial. For example, pushing people out of a plane without a parachute to see if they live or die vs. allowing them to stay in the plane and land safely, would not require a large sample size. About ten, probably... any volunteers?

However, as the effects become smaller and smaller, you need to recruit more and more people to pick up a significant difference. If you think the difference is really quite small, you need thousands of volunteers to be studied, over many years.

At this point my argument is pretty straightforward. If you really feel that you need to treat 10,000 people, over 5 years, in order to show any significant benefit, then that benefit is likely to be so small as to be not worth bothering about. I think this is a pretty good principle.

Of course, fellow medics and researchers will howl in incandescent rage at this statement. But I think I stand by it. For you will find that, when we enter the world of statistical significance, the figures themselves can be extremely... shall we say, disappointing.

I first became aware of this with the first major trial on lowering blood pressure. As with many medical interventions, lowering blood pressure was considered such a wonderful thing that no clinical study had been reported on lowering 'mild' hypertension, until the mid-1980s.[29]

I should mention that mild hypertension, at that time, was a diastolic blood pressure of 90-109 mmHg. Nowadays, if you had a diastolic of 109 mmHg, you would virtually be rushed into hospital with malignant hypertension – as I have said before – my how definitions change.

This was the Medical Research Council (MRC) study, and the main aim of the trial was to determine whether drug treatment of mild hypertension in men and women aged 35-64 years reduced the rates of:

- Stroke

- Death due to hypertension

- Coronary events

17,354 patients were recruited and split into two equal groups. The trials lasted a bit over five years which means that there were 85,572 patient years of observation. Which is a lot of people, and a lot of years. And here are the results in absolute figures.

	BP lowering medication	Placebo
Fatal strokes	18	27
Fatal Coronary events	106	97
Stroke + myocardial infarction (MI) deaths	124	124
Deaths	248	253

As you can see, after all this time, on all these patients, the difference in the rate of death due to stroke and heart attacks (MIs) was exactly and precisely zero. There were five more deaths in the placebo arm due to five more deaths from abdominal aneurysm rupture (which could possibly be an effect of raised blood pressure).

What effect did this have on the ongoing and active treatment of mild hypertension? As you would expect. None at all.

However, the main point of bringing up this trial again is to highlight how small the absolute figures can be, yet produce headlines such as: *"MRC study demonstrates that lowering mild blood pressure results in a 33% reduction in fatal strokes".*

Yes, after stripping this area to its very bones, the authors of this study managed to find statistical significance when they looked at one of the drugs used vs. the other in stroke. A difference of 9 deaths: 18 versus 27, in 17,354 patients, over 5 years, can be, somehow or another, turned into something that is statistically significant.

In short, when a trial announces with a great fanfare that overall mortality was significantly reduced on treatment, you may now have some idea of how minute, in absolute figures, that difference can be. In a similar vein, you now also have some idea of how vanishingly small any difference in overall mortality has to be, for it *not* to show up at all i.e. women and statins.

So, when someone states that their trial was 'not adequately powered' to demonstrate a reduction in mortality, you have to ask yourself just how small was the improvement they were expecting to find?

For example, to look at a completely theoretical study. If you did a study with 5,000 people taking a placebo, and 5,000 taking a drug of some sort, and you expected a mortality rate of 2% in the placebo arm, then you would achieve statistical significance if *twenty* fewer people died in the treatment arm. Probability $p < 0.045$.

20 fewer people dead, out of 5,000, after 5 years; and that, ladies and gentlemen, would be statistically significant. If you were looking for this difference at the start, you could then say that your study was sufficiently powered at the outset.

Of course, if you don't think you are going to show any significant effect on overall mortality you can also choose not to 'power' it for this end-point before the study starts. Instead you power it to look for other end-points e.g. number of strokes prevented (fatal, or non-fatal), number of hospital admissions prevented.

At this point we move into the 'heads I win, tails you lose', game. If the trial were not adequately 'powered' before it starts then the investigators will dismiss a lack of impact on overall mortality as, *'exactly what you would expect, as this trial was not powered to detect a difference.'*

On the other hand, if there were an impact on overall mortality they will do a post-hoc analysis – and trumpet a positive effect (as per MRC study on mild hypertension). Now, you are not supposed to do this. If you didn't power the study properly, you didn't power the study properly, and you can't claim you did if you get a better than expected result. But researchers do this all the time. I believe that this game is constantly played, but I have no evidence. Getting to see the pre-trial statistical criteria has been, basically, impossible. I am told that statistical analysis reports are now being made available, but I have not come across many in the public domain.

I feel that this is probably enough on overall mortality and the games that are played with it – and around it. As with many things in this world, the concept of overall mortality sounds very simple at first. However, when you start looking into it, it rapidly becomes a complicated and slippery customer.

The main take-away messages are, just as a reminder, as follows:

- If overall mortality isn't mentioned, then overall mortality was unchanged;

- If you hear this type of phrase 'overall mortality from heart disease was significantly reduced,' then overall mortality was unchanged;

- If someone says a study was not powered to detect an effect on overall morality, then overall mortality was unchanged;

- If overall mortality was unchanged, then whatever else is being said is highly unlikely to matter very much for your health.

Cancer Screening & risk

Earlier on I did praise the world of cancer for being clear about one thing. Rather than using concepts such as lives saved, or relative risk reduction in death, researchers in this area tend to look at increase in survival time i.e. how much longer are you are likely to live for, if you take this treatment. This is good.

However, when it comes to cancer screening rather than cancer treatments, we enter a very different world indeed. Whilst risk is happily distorted and mangled throughout medical research, it probably reaches its apogee in cancer screening, where it can be nearly impossible to understand what the statistics mean. In some cases, absolutely impossible, or maybe that's just me.

As chance would have it, at almost exactly the same time as I was starting to write this chapter, someone sent me an e-mail with a link to a study called "Do Physicians Understand Cancer Screening Statistics? A National Survey of Primary Care Physicians in the United States."[30] This paper came to the following, extremely important, conclusions:

"Physicians clearly do not understand how to interpret cancer screening statistics."
"It is natural to assume that survival is the same as mortality; that is what the words imply in common language."

The first quote here sounds a bit damning of the medical profession, but it merely confirms what has become increasingly clear to me.

Namely, that cancer screening statistics are impenetrable, and incomprehensible, even to doctors. And if doctors can't understand this stuff, when they are supposed to have been trained in the area, what chance for the average member of the public? (0.0025% probably).

The second quote is more complex. *"It is natural to assume that survival is the same as mortality; that is what the words imply in common language."* However, I will attempt to explain what it means later, as it represents a critical point.

Starting with the crude interpretation of cancer statistics, here is the commentary on one part of the study "Do Physicians Understand Cancer Screening Statistics." Doctors were asked to look at a hypothetical screening test (in reality it was prostate cancer screening). They were told that the 5-year survival rate improved from 68% to 99% if men were screened. The result of this is that...

"Many of the physicians appear to have mistakenly interpreted survival in screening as if it were survival in the context of a treatment trial, note the authors. After reviewing only the 5-year survival rates in the scenario provided (99% vs 68%), almost half the respondents who thought that 'lives were saved' stated that there would be 300 to 310 fewer cancer deaths per 1000 people screened."[31]

I suppose that most people, if they were told that 5-year survival rate improved by 30%, would assume that this would result in 300 (or thereabouts) fewer cancer deaths for every 1,000 people screened. As this appears to be what these words mean. Indeed, how could they possibly mean anything else?

However, if we continue looking at this paper, we find that:

"The actual reduction in cancer mortality demonstrated in the European Randomized Study of Screening for Prostate Cancer was about 0.4 in 1000 within 5 years."

You may be thinking, how do you get from 99% vs 68% cure rate, to a 0.4 per 1,000 per 5 years? And how can both figures be correct? As you may have guessed this is primarily a situation whereby we are being presented with relative risks massaged to look like absolute risks. With a whole bunch of extra added twists...

(At this point I need to add that although I am talking about prostate cancer screening here, this does not mean that the absolute figures are the same in various papers on the subject. So, as I run through the figures, do not expect them to end up at 0.4 per 1,000 per 5 years. No two papers on this subject agree on figures – for a myriad of reasons that I am leaving well alone here. I am just highlighting general principles at this point).

First, looking at relative risks.

The number of new cases of prostate cancer detected per year in the UK, (known as the incidence rate) is 97.2 per 100,000 (or 0.972 per 1,000). Which broadly means that if you screened 1,000 men each year, very slightly fewer than 1 could be diagnosed as having prostate cancer[iv].

This means that, even if your screening test were perfect, you could only pick up 1 man for every 1,000 screened because that's how many men have new/undiagnosed prostate cancer out there in the community (At this point, let's go back to the 97 men in 100,000 and let's make the maths simple and say that there are 100 men in 100,000 who would show signs of prostate cancer if screened, or 1 in 1,000).

Looking at this the other way round. You screen 1,000 men. You can pick up 1 with prostate cancer (assuming your test is perfect). If 99% of them survive five years, this is 0.99 per thousand, or 0.099%.

If cancer appears through symptoms, there will be a 0.68 per thousand survival rate. Or 0.068%. The difference between 0.099 and 0.068 is 0.031. (Or 0.3 per thousand).

Very quickly, by looking at absolute instead of relative risk, we reduce the numbers potentially 'cured' by screening from 300 per 1,000 to 0.3 per 1,000. Which would obviously come as a major surprise to the majority of doctors who managed to overestimate the benefit of screening by a factor of 1,000. Not bad going guys. Repeat after me, '0.03 multiplied by 1 is *not* 300'.

Of course things don't stop here. At this point we have to factor in the knowledge that the vast majority of men diagnosed with prostate cancer do not die of it, they die *with* it. Prostate cancer is often a very slow growing cancer that sits about doing very little. If you diagnosed it in an 80 year old, very often the best thing to do is... nothing.

Then, of course, you have to take into account that screening will never happen yearly, that your test is not perfect, that some men will never turn up for screening, and the maximum possible benefits of screening begin to get smaller and smaller. Eventually shrinking down to 0.4 per 1,000 per 5 years (or somewhere in that ball park).

---

iv Assuming your test was perfect, and also assuming a lot of other things about the PSA test that are far from certain. And assuming a whole other series of things about pre-test probabilities etc.

What is survival anyway?

Unfortunately, once you do strip the figures down into their component parts, the complications do not end. In cancer screening a further massive element of confusion is lobbed into the ring.

Which is that the word survival does **not** mean that you will actually survive. To quote again from the paper on physicians understanding of cancer screening again... *"It is natural to assume that survival is the same as mortality; that is what the words imply in common language."*

"When I use a word," Humpty Dumpty said in rather a scornful tone, "it means just what I choose it to mean – neither more nor less."

"The question is," said Alice, "whether you can make words mean so many different things."

"The question is," said Humpty Dumpty, "which is to be master – that's all."

In the world of cancer screening the term 'survival' is taken to mean that you are still alive five years after the cancer was first diagnosed. Five year cancer survival rate is the measure used for almost all interventions in this area. Or to turn this around slightly, if you survive for five years after your initial cancer diagnosis, the statisticians will consider that you have been cured.

As a result of this, if a screening test picks up cancer five years earlier than would have happened, had it appeared through symptoms, the five-year survival/cure will automatically appear to be astronomically better. Especially with a slow growing cancer (such as prostate).

Even if you did absolutely nothing at all after detecting the cancer, you will improve the 'cure rate' to very nearly 100%, as almost everyone will survive for at least five years after the initial diagnosis. Apart from those who get hit by a bus, or die as their brain bursts during a vain attempt to understand medical statistics

Words, words, words, words, words. They really should mean something. So should medical statistics but they don't. Or their meaning is so wildly distorted that even doctors cannot understand the figures they are looking at. Which is a bit disturbing, as doctors are usually the people that other people go to when they have questions about medical care.

Not the blind leading the blind, but perhaps the horribly confused leading the even more horribly confused?

Patient: 'Doctor, should I be screened for prostate cancer?'

Doctor: 'Absolutely, you will reduce your risk of dying by over 30%...

by the way, would you like a cup of tea that I have just made in my brand new chocolate teapot?'

All of this is not, I firmly believe, a form of absent-minded carelessness. Much of it is quite deliberate. There are many people with an agenda out there, and they will ruthlessly torture statistics until they get the answer they want out of them.

"Difficulty is a coin the learned make use of, like jugglers, to conceal the inanity of their art."

Michel de Montaigne

Those involved in cancer screening have even created their own, virtually-impossible-to-understand language, in order to make their figures look stunning. Stunning they may look, but luckily there are other people out there who are less than stunned, and who choose to look a bit more closely.

The United States Preventative Task force reviewed all the data on Prostate Cancer screening (using the prostate specific antigen (P.S.A.) blood test) and came to the conclusion that it does more harm than good.

*"**U.S. Panel Says No to Prostate Screening for Healthy Men**. Healthy men should no longer receive a P.S.A. blood test to screen for prostate cancer because the test does not save lives overall and often leads to more tests and treatments that needlessly cause pain, impotence and incontinence in many, a key government health panel has decided."* [32]

Lo, it turns out that the prostate screening test, which improves survival from 68% to 99% does not actually save lives – at all. Fantastic sounding cure rates, which completely bedazzle doctors, are simply meaningless.

Women shall be saved too

Despite this, all statistics on cancer screening continue to be presented in the most optimistic and skeptic crushing manner. Here, for example, is a headline that appeared on the BBC news site on cervical cancer. It was the first one that appeared as I started researching, and writing, this chapter.

"Women diagnosed with cervical cancer as a result of a smear test have a far better chance of being cured than women who do not go for tests, a Swedish study suggests. The researchers found a 92% cure rate after a smear test diagnosis, compared with 66% for symptoms-based diagnoses." [33]

Oh goody, I thought. 92% vs 66% cure rates. How amazing! Not quite as good as prostate cancer screening, but never mind. On the face of it, this appears to represent an absolute risk reduction of 26%. Or, turning this around, if you have a smear there is a 425% relative increase in the chance of a cure (34% vs. 8% not cured).

Things could not look much better than this could they? So surely women must have regular smear tests to protect themselves from dying of cervical cancer. To do otherwise is madness, madness I tell you.

Well, to be truthful, I did not actually think these things. What I really thought was. Oh, bloody hell, here we go again. Yet another study I am going to have to read and try to understand what they did, and how they did it. More tortured prose, more opaque statistical tests, more assumptions made that I will have to try to track down... aaarrrgh! Have pity on my poor brain.

Of course, before reading the paper I knew a couple of things to start with. First, if 1,000 women have a smear this is **not** going to stop 260 from dying of cervical cancer. Secondly, the word cure will **not** mean cure – at least not in the sense that the vast majority of people would understand. Reading that last sentence I think I am gradually turning into a rather thick version of Emmanuel Kant.

Anyway, moving on, this study was published in the BMJ, so you most likely cannot access it, as they charge for looking at research nowadays. However, if you do have access, here it is.[34] As a member of the BMA I get free access to all articles. I can also access almost all other medical journals as well...

The first thing to note about this study was that it was an observational study. In the author's own words:

"Randomised controlled trials are not feasible for the evaluation of established cervical screening programmes, which is why the only alternative is well designed observational studies."

As I hope to have made clear earlier on, it is not possible to prove causality with observational studies. I would also like to make it clear that you cannot state that the only 'alternative' to an interventional study is a well-designed observational study.

A well-designed observational study cannot be considered an *alternative* to an interventional study. This disingenuous phrase implies that the two things are in some way comparable. When they are not, even remotely. The statement should read:

'Unfortunately randomised controlled trials are not feasible for the evaluation of established cervical screening programmes, so we have to rely on far weaker sources of evidence which are subject to many confounders and other sources of bias i.e. observational studies like this rather shoddy one.'

Indeed, when it comes to cancer screening there is a well-established 'built-in' problem with bias. For it is well known that women who attend regularly for screening tend to be of higher social status, more highly educated, more health conscious, more... well, healthy.

As the authors of the study admit: *"A healthy volunteer bias or health selection does not seem to explain our findings, although an effect of confounding cannot be ruled out."*

You're damned right that an effect confounding cannot be ruled out. See under Hormone Replacement Therapy to prevent cardio vascular disease. However, as I suspect now becomes wearisomely familiar, the fact that this was an observational study does not appear in any press release. All we get is the usual triumphant blast of non-critical hype. The BBC article contained the following commentary

"Robert Music, director of Jo's Cervical Cancer Trust, said the research highlighted the importance of attending cervical screening. 'Cervical cancer is largely preventable thanks to cervical screening which saves 5,000 UK lives a year. And for those diagnosed, survival rates are good if the disease is caught early.

"There is an urgent need for more investment in targeted campaigns to remind women that they can take proactive steps to reduce their risk of cervical cancer by attending screening. Quite simply it could save their life.'"

No caution here, not even a hint of caution. We even get my favorite phrase 'life saving' thrown in twice for good measure.

The reality is that there has never been a randomised controlled study on the benefits of cervical cancer screening done anywhere – ever. As with most forms of screening, it was introduced using the well-established scientific principle that '*a stitch in time saves nine.*'

I suppose most people probably believe that universal cancer screening programmes must have been introduced on the back of rigorous clinical studies. Well, think again. Cancer screening has generally been thought to be such an obviously good thing that the very idea it might require scientific validation was never really considered. After all 'prevention is better than cure,' is it not?

Of course, none of this means that it is not a good thing to do – it might well be. But you cannot get round the elephant in the room which is that, once you have started trying to screen everybody it becomes virtually impossible to prove that screening works – or does not work.

For the very simple reason that any attempt at randomisation has just been thrown out of the window. Where is our control arm if everyone is being screened? You're right, you cannot have one. After you have introduced universal screening programmes you have to pray that they really do work, because you will never again have a real opportunity to prove that they do.

People have tried to find some evidence to support cervical cancer screening by looking to see if the overall death rate from cervical cancer fell after screening first started in around the mid-1960s. Did the rate of cervical cancer plummet, or rise?

Sadly, these data do not really tell us anything one way or another. Since 1971 cervical cancer rates have certainly fallen dramatically. On the face of it, this seems to strongly support the idea that screening has been highly beneficial.

However, deaths from cervical cancer have fallen most rapidly in the 75-85 age group (where no screening has ever taken place) than in the 25-44 age group, where screening is done most frequently. In fact, cervical cancer deaths in the younger age group went up, then down, then up, then down, and are now basically flat. What interpretation would you like to make of those facts?

You would be a brave man to claim causality – although this is exactly what people do when they state things such as...'thanks to cervical cancer screening which saves 5,000 lives a year.' Once again, please note the use of the concept of live saving, then repeat after me one hundred times. 'You cannot save a life, all you can do is delay death.'

However, without getting dragged too far into the mire of population statistics and the impossibility of doing a randomised controlled trial in this area, when I finally gathered the energy to read this paper I found it rapidly becoming stranger and stranger – and considerably more difficult to understand.

The first problem was that, although it was reported that 1,230 women were diagnosed with cervical cancer, when I looked at the figures in more detail, I found the following:

Screen detected cancers	=	273
Symptomatic cancers	=	567
Total	=	840

This was a study purportedly on 1,230 women diagnosed with cervical cancer. However, as far I could ascertain, it seemed to have only 840 women in it. 390 women had gone missing. This type of thing happens in medical papers all the time. Which leaves you playing the scientific equivalent of 'Where's Wally?' I knew the missing 390 had to be somewhere, but finding them was different matter.

There was no mention of the missing 390 in: the abstract; the introduction; and the discussion. Which are the only bits I generally read, and are also the bits that are supposed to give a good overview of the entire paper. You would think that if one third of your study population had been excluded from the analysis, this would at least merit some sort of a comment as to why it had been done.

Maybe I have become a bit paranoid about things like this. 'Does it really matter?' You might exclaim. Well, it matters that you have to spend two hours of your valuable life searching for this elusive group, then trying to work out where they went. It also matters in that it is scientifically dishonest. You claim your study is on 1,230 women, but it is not. It is on 840 women.

As it turns out the explanation was simple. 390 women were too old to be included in the main analysis, as they were above the age where screening stops. Fair enough you might think, but why didn't they just say this somewhere ? It only took me 21 words to explain it.

Perhaps most significantly, amongst the 390 'excluded' women there were 196 of the total deaths from cervical cancer vs. 176 in the those of screening age. A figure that represents 53% of the total number of cervical cancer deaths. This could otherwise be expressed as... a majority.

Why then, did they continue to mention 1,230 women, and 373 deaths throughout the paper when this was actually an analysis of 840 women and 176 deaths? I leave the explanation up to you, but I know what I think.

Mind you, having tracked down the missing 390, my comprehension difficulties had only just started. Cervical cancer screening is normally supposed to happen every three years. So, you would think the main comparison in this study would be between women who had a smear every three years vs. women who had never had a smear, or who only turned up every so often for a smear.

But no.

The main comparison here was between women who had a smear between one and six months before a diagnosis of cervical cancer was made, and all other women (including those who regularly turned up for a smear) who presented to their doctor with symptoms.

By creating this 'virtual' group of women, it is not exactly amazing to find that those who had cervical cancer diagnosed through a smear test are going to do better than those who present with symptoms – as they are almost certainly going to have an earlier stage cancer detected.

Or, to put this another way, their cancer was diagnosed, on average, a couple of years earlier than those who presented with symptoms – so five year survival had to be improved by at least two years (see previous section). This issue *was* noted by the authors, but it was covered by the following opaque sentence: *"One limitation of cure models is that they estimate a cure proportion even when statistical cure is not reached."*

A sentence which, I suspect would have meant absolutely nothing to you before reading this far. However, now you know what it means. It means that the word cure does not actually mean cure – in any sense that most people in the world would understand it. Also, that diagnosing cancer earlier will automatically skew five year survival figures in favour of screening.

If you want to claim that a screening programme has benefits you need to match those who are 'regularly' screened vs. those who are not. This will give you a true idea of the possible benefits of any actual programme that actually exists in the real world.

You cannot just create a 'virtual' group of women, then make claims as to how much this group would benefit were they to manage, somehow or other, to have a smear test six months before cervical cancer would have appeared. There is no such group. They are a statistical chimera.

If, instead of using this artificially created population, we look at two groups that are based in reality; those who were regularly screened vs. those not screened, then the figures undergo a rapid and dramatic change. The 26% benefit immediately contracts to 8% (82 vs 74% 'cure' rate). And yes, these figures are in the paper – parked away, and not at all easy to find.

I realise that this has all got rather detailed, and complex, and requires a lot of concentration. However, I believe that explaining this type of statistical mangling is really important in helping us to take control of data doctoring.

Let's take stock as to where we have reached at this point.

- Although the abstract, discussion, and conclusions of this paper state that this was a study of 1,230 women, and 373 deaths. It was, in reality, a study of 840 women and 176 deaths – in women of screening ages.

- Although the authors claimed a 26% reduction in cervical cancers in those screened, this figure comes from a group of women that do not exist in real life, unless the screening interval is going to be reduced from three years to six months (which was not done in this study, and is not done anywhere in the world).

- The relative risk reduction in those screened regularly vs. those not screened regularly/ not screened at all, was actually 8%.

What you also need to keep sharply in focus at this point is that, so far, I have just been talking about *relative* differences in 'cure', not absolute numbers. In order to establish the absolute risk reduction we have to know how many women were included in this study in the first place.

This figure was not mentioned anywhere in the paper, so I had to do a bit of my own research on the matter. I knew that this was an analysis of all women of screening age in Sweden i.e. those between the ages 20 and 60. This, I discovered, represents a total population of very nearly 2,500,000 women.

What this means is that out of a 2,500,000 women, 840 were diagnosed with cervical cancer and 176 died of cervical cancer. A smaller proportion than you might have imagined. I imagine.

Next, we need to look at the total number of deaths in those screened vs. those not screened/irregularly screened:

- Regularly screened 71 deaths (out of 431 diagnosed cases)

- Not screened/irregularly screened 106 deaths (out of 409 diagnosed cases)

- Total difference = 35

Which means that, over 3 years, in a potential screening population of 2,500,000 women, 35 cases of cervical cancer might have been 'cured'. Yes, that is correct, 35 women out of 2,500,000. Or, approximately 1 in 70,000. Better odds than winning the lottery, I suppose. This assumes the study was not biased by 'healthy volunteer' effect, i.e. Women who look after themselves are more likely to be screened.

I suppose this rather begs the question, why do people play these complicated games? I suppose we all want to convince ourselves that what we are doing is fantastically beneficial. We don't want naysayers, we don't want criticism. This is just basic human nature. We all want to prevent cancer, and save men and women from dying.

In addition, the underlying concept of cancer screening is seductively simple. Pick up cancer very early, then cure it. This must be beneficial, it just MUST be. Well, maybe it is, maybe not. Don't get me wrong I am not against screening altogether.

In fact I have a favorite screening test. It is simply to take someone's pulse. You can tell within about ten seconds if they have atrial fibrillation. If they do, you can prescribe an anticoagulant, and reduce the risk of stroke (relative) by 40%.

A simple non-invasive test that costs nothing to do. It picks up a condition for which there is an effective treatment. There is no downside, no unintentional harm to the patient. Of course, there is no screening programme for atrial fibrillation in place anywhere in the world. Go figure.

However, to return to the main theme of this chapter, which is all about the games that are played with risk, and screening designed to reduce risk. If I can summarise, it would to make three points:

1. Relative vs. Absolute risk. Relative figures are usually presented as though they are absolute. This results in the benefits of screening looking as if they are hundreds, thousands, even hundreds of thousands of times more impressive than they actually are.

2. Cure does not mean cure. A problem unique to this area is that the word 'cure' does not actually mean cure. It means the number who survive five years after diagnosis, usually in cancer. This means that, in the case of very slow growing cancers e.g. prostate, five year survival is virtually guaranteed to reach almost 100% if you pick up the cancer five years earlier.

3. The studies have not been done. Perhaps the greatest problem in this whole area is that most cancer screening programmes were started without anyone having first done a randomised controlled study. This makes it exceedingly difficult to prove that a cancer screening programme has any benefit at all, as there is no way to do a randomised study ever again.

The JUPITER trial

Moving out of cancer, and back to heart disease. Sometimes a trial appears that is so perfectly incomprehensible it can take months to work out what has just been said. Which takes me to the JUPITER study. JUPITER stands for... **J**ustification for the **U**se of Statins in **P**rimary Prevention: An **I**ntervention **T**rial **E**valuating **R**osuvastatin trial (acronyms away lads).

All cardiovascular studies done by the pharmaceutical company AstraZeneca have a theme of space. There is METEOR, SATURN, STELLAR, AURORA, CORONA and suchlike. No doubt a marketing company charged them $100 million for this cunning bit of branding – so effective that I can guarantee you never even noticed. Money well spent, I say.

This study was considered so significant that it terminated early. Such were the observed benefits, that it was considered unethical to continue giving a placebo to those who could benefit from the statin. Here were the headline findings:

"'Compared to those who received placebo, patients receiving the drug rosuvastatin had a 48% reduction in stroke, a 46% reduction in the need for interventions to reopen blocked blood vessels, and a 20% drop in all cause mortality,' said Paul Ridker, the study's lead author."[35]

The sheer magnificence of these results was re-iterated by Steven Nissen, a highly influential research cardiologist.

"'The extent of reduction in death, heart attacks, and stroke is larger than we've seen in any trial I can remember,' said Dr Steven Nissen, a prominent Cleveland Clinic cardiologist. 'I don't know how you get much bigger than that.'"[36]

All hail JUPITER!

You might be thinking, at this point. What is incomprehensible about those results? After all, the study was stopped early due to the vast scale of the benefits. Secondly, there was a 20% drop in all-cause mortality. All-cause mortality means dying of anything. Another term for this would be – death, or being dead.

Surely, after what I have said earlier, this is a good thing. All-cause mortality is the most simple and certain to measure end-point. If 20% more people were alive in the statin arm at the end of the study this was surely a good thing. Well, it would be a very good thing if that is actually what it meant.

The 20% drop was of course a *relative* reduction in mortality and re-member what I have already said about relative anything. The absolute reduction was rather different. At the risk of inducing a deep sleep, I will go through the figures:

There were 8,901 people in the placebo arm at the start of the trial, and another 8,901 in the statin arm. The number of those dying in each arm was 235/8,901 vs. 190/8,901...

Which is 2.64% vs. 2.14%

An absolute difference of 0.5%

This could also be represented as NNT = 200 over the 2 years of treatment. (NNT 400 for 1 year).

If you want to see this in graphical form, here it is.[37] The two graphs here are actually just different versions of each other. The upper right hand graph represents a highly magnified version of the bigger graph.

Expanded like this you can actually see that the two mortality lines start to move back together, just after four years have passed. Gosh, that was happening at the exact time that the trial was stopped... what a strange coincidence. Who'd have believed it... you don't think... etc.

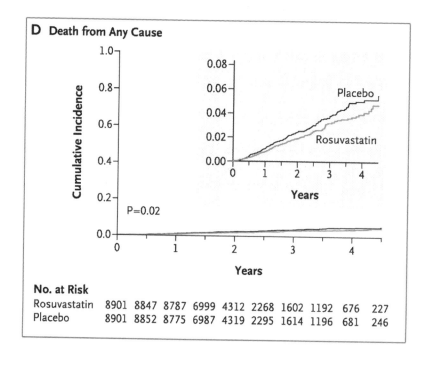

(You could ask, how come the graph covers four years, when the study was stopped after an average of less than two. That is because people started the trial at different times, any more explanation than this and complicated equations must follow).

Anyway, to quote Steven Nissen "*I don't know how you get much bigger than that.*" Ah yes, gentle reader, cardiologists are clearly an easily impressed bunch. They also use very thin pens to draw lines, or you would not be able to discern any difference between the placebo line, and the rosuvastatin line, in the main graph.

However, to get back to the main point. What was incomprehensible about this study? Well, in order to answer this, I have to establish some context.

Statin trials have been, essentially, divided into two types. The first type was done on people who had already suffered from a stroke, or heart attack, or such-like. It was hoped that the statin would 'prevent' a second event. Which is why they are referred to as secondary prevention trials.

Secondary prevention trials up to now have shown a reduction in the risk of further strokes and heart attacks in both men and women. They have also demonstrated a reduction in overall mortality in men, but not in women. About 5% of the adult population would be considered suitable for secondary prevention. Secondary prevention meaning that they already have some form of diagnosed cardiovascular disease.

On the other hand, primary prevention studies were done to look at those who did not have any (yet diagnosed), cardiovascular disease. Until Jupiter came along, primary prevention studies had managed to show a reduction in cardiovascular mortality in men, but not in women. However, and this is critical. No primary prevention study had ever shown a reduction in overall mortality – dying of any cause – in either men or women.

This had acted as a bit of a barrier to the take-up of statins in primary prevention. With no overall mortality benefit, it was difficult to argue that any cardiovascular benefits outweighed costs, added workload, and the potential adverse effects of the drugs themselves.

So the stage was set for a primary prevention study to demonstrate a benefit on overall mortality. This would clear away any objections to using statins in a much bigger market. Basically, all living adults with a cholesterol level above zero.

When you consider that a single statin, Lipitor (atorvastatin) was already making £13 billion per year for Pfizer, in a more restricted market, you can see that the sums of money involved were eye-watering.

And lo it came to pass that the JUPITER study did exactly what was required. It showed a significant impact on overall mortality. The potential financial effect of this was outlined in the *BMJ* by Professor John Abramson of Harvard University:

"This study may have the greatest effect on the cost and delivery of medicine of any study that has ever been published," he said. *"It is going to substantially increase the costs of health care."*

This held true despite the fact that the absolute change in mortality was considerably less stunning than the headlines would have us believe. You had to treat 400 people for 1 year to delay 1 death. But, to be fair, statistical significance is statistical significance. Five toes above the water in the bath. (Look it up).

In addition, as mentioned earlier, overall mortality is a pretty powerful, robust and clear-cut end-point. Someone is either dead, or they are not. You can hardly pretend… 'Quick, hold your breath for five minutes, and I can record you as dead.' Equally, you would struggle to make dead people look lively. Other end-points, such as hospitalisation, are more open to, shall we say, interpretation.

If there were potential problems with these data, where could they be? I thank Professor Michel de Lorgeril for pointing them out. Because, at first, I couldn't see them at all, although they were staring me in the face. Typical of a man looking for anything, so I am told by someone living not a million miles away from me.

The main problem goes like this:

Statins were developed to stop people dying of cardiovascular disease. Heart attacks and strokes mainly. They have not been shown to reduce deaths from any other cause – ever. Therefore, one would expect that if there were a reduction in overall mortality, it would have to be due to a reduction in cardiovascular deaths. Would it not?

On this basis, the JUPITER trials started off pretty well. If you look at the total number of heart attacks, there were 31 in the statin arm, and 68 in the placebo arm. Relatively speaking, there were more than twice as many heart attacks in the placebo arm.

However, and please read this bit slowly. There were 22 *non-fatal* MIs in the statin arm, and 62 *non-fatal* MIs in the placebo arm.

I shall put this another way:

- In those taking the statin there were thirty one heart attacks which resulted in nine deaths.

- In those taking a placebo there were sixty eight heart attacks which resulted in six deaths.

If we look at stroke:

- In those taking a statin there were thirty three strokes resulting in three deaths.

- In those taking a placebo there were sixty four strokes resulting in six deaths.

If we add heart attacks to stroke, we find that:

- In the statin arm there were twelve deaths from stroke and heart attacks.

- In the placebo arm there were twelve deaths from stroke and heart attacks.

It does not take the use of a super-computer to work out that the difference between twelve, and twelve, is zero. Although it did take a bit of detective work to establish these figures.

To quote Michel de Lorgeril, in the rather damning article he wrote in the *Archives of Internal Medicine*:

"Although it is quite unusual that the burden of calculating cardiovascular mortality is placed on the readers, all methods used, however, lead to the same conclusion: there is no significant difference in cardiovascular mortality between the 2 groups in the JUPITER trial."[38]

The lead author, Paul Ridker, came back with some highly scientific criticism of the criticism. Including such gems as these:

"In this world, no matter how clear and blue the sky is, there will always be people who look up and see nothing but rain."

"It's okay with me if these physicians want to ignore the data. I just don't want them taking care of my patients or my family."

And my personal favorite:

"This is more evidence that Europe doesn't really want to prevent heart disease."[39]

Naughty Europe, I say. Whoever, or whatever, Europe may actually be. Luckily, I am British, so I am not part of Europe at all. In fact, as a Scotsman, I denounce Europe and its callous wish to see all of its citizens drop dead of heart disease. That's socialised medicine for you, I suppose.

Anyway, once you hack through the deep dark statistical 'jungle of obfuscation', it turns out that any difference in deaths was primarily due to far fewer deaths from cancer in those taking the statin. Something seen in no other statin study, ever. Hmmmm, a drug that can cause a significant reduction in cancer deaths, in under two years. All this when five year long statin studies, with far more patients in them, have not seen any beneficial effect on cancer.

I am not even going to go into how ridiculous it would be to claim this could be a real effect. [v] Let's just say, if you threw a dice twice, and got two sixes, this would be far less likely than the probability of this result. Did someone shout chance? I suppose it is better than shouting the alternative word.

To my mind, the main lesson of the JUPITER study is that we have now reached a point where the true findings of a study are so carefully spun that it can be almost impossible to establish what was found. No-one is lying but, by golly, they are getting mightily close.

"Compared to those who received placebo, patients receiving the drug rosuvastatin had a 48% reduction in stroke, a 46% reduction in the need for interventions to reopen blocked blood vessels, and a 20% drop in all cause mortality.
"The extent of reduction in death, heart attacks, and stroke is larger than we've seen in any trial I can remember," said Dr Steven Nissen.

If you read these two statements, I have no doubt what you are supposed to think. That rosuvastatin reduced cardiovascular mortality by a very significant amount. So much so, that it even managed to reduce all-cause mortality. (It requires bigger numbers/effects to show an impact on dying of everything, rather than just one thing).

---

v Dr Uffe Ravnskov explains this well – cholesterol is healthful and protective. People with high cholesterol have lower incidence of cancer, but are also more likely to be put on statins. De Facto – people on statins have lower cancer rates.

When, what it actually showed was that rosuvastatin had no impact on fatal heart attacks, or strokes, and the effect on overall mortality was primarily due to a drop in cancer deaths (58 placebo vs 35 rosuvastatin). As for where the other deaths went... it is absolutely impossible to work this out. Death due to dying, perhaps.

Summary of risk – the eight point check list

If I can try to summarise things in this area, I would give the following advice:

- Most risk is presented as a relative risk – which can make small risks sound terrifying or reduction in the risk unbelievably good.

- Most benefits are presented as relative – which greatly inflates perceived benefit.

- You should always try to establish the absolute change in risk or benefit.

- When someone says they can reduce the risk of death – they are talking rubbish.

- If you cannot understand what is being said – this may well be deliberate.

- If you cannot understand what is being said – it probably doesn't matter anyway.

- Look for impact on mortality/life expectancy – if you cannot find it, it means there was no impact.

- The most important measure is increased, or reduced, life expectancy.

CHAPTER FOUR

Things that are not true
are often held to be true

My main area of interest for the last 30 years has been cardiovascular disease, and so I know it better than any other. Possibly the most fascinating, and disturbing, thing to emerge, to my mind at least, is the existence of a whole series of 'facts', which are just not true. Or, to be somewhat more scientific in my use of language, they are facts with no clinical outcome evidence to support them. Here is one such 'fact', which is very widely accepted as true: red wine protects against heart disease.

When you try to track down a fact like this you will find that the evidence it rests on varies from weak, to nil, to completely contradictory. Indeed, if you have the time and energy required to dig deeper, you will find that most such facts are not based on any data at all. It can simply be an idea that was put forward in a medical journal, or at a conference by someone. Sometimes it is impossible to find the source – it just seems to have emerged from the ether.

Despite the lack of any scientific foundation, a strange thing then happens to certain ideas. Over time, through a process of repetition, and multiple cross-referencing between different authors, and journals, the initial hypothesis becomes widely accepted as being true. How and why? Because everyone says... that everyone else says it is true.

There will almost always be some physiological or biochemical process invoked to give it some scientific credibility of some sort. But when you look for the real hard data on clinical outcomes... nothing.

The female paradox

The first time I came across an example of this phenomenon was when I started looking more closely at the 'fact' that women were protected against heart disease by their sex hormones. At one point this was so widely believed to be true that I didn't even bother to question it. After all, younger women had (and still have) far lower rates of heart disease than men. However, when women reach the menopause, their rate of heart disease explodes... does it not?

In reality it does not. Or, to be more accurate, the rise in the rate of CHD in women represents a smooth accelerating upward curve which perfectly matches an increase in age, and is totally unaffected by the menopause. In most populations it lags behind the mortality curve of men by about ten years – for complex reasons that I am not going to discuss here.

I did not know this at the time. Like almost everyone else, I believed what I had been told, and I was interested in finding out exactly how women were protected.

At first I believed that finding the mechanism would be simple. Somewhere, I would find *the* major study proving that oestrogen and progesterone (UK spelling) had beneficial effects. However, after a frustrating and prolonged search (this took place in a time long before the Internet) I found no evidence at all. I came to understand that the reason why I could not find it was because it DID NOT EXIST.

There had been some work done on rabbits in the 1950s, which seemed to show that rabbit female sex hormones had some beneficial effect on cholesterol levels. A couple of snippets showed that oestrogen lowered LDL and raised HDL, a bit, and that was pretty much all there was.

To my surprise (I would be completely unsurprised today), no-one had ever done a study on humans, and no controlled clinical trial existed. The entire 'wealth' of research into this area resembled a vast barren desert, with a few tumbleweed blowing in the wind.

Despite the complete lack of any foundations, by around the early 1960s the female sex hormone hypothesis was being presented in scientific conferences and medical papers in terms that brooked no argument on the matter. It was just true, end of discussion. The idea gathered an almost unstoppable momentum.

Adding to this, a study was done in 1987, which appeared to prove conclusively that Hormone Replacement Therapy (HRT) was indeed highly protective against CVD. A study I mentioned earlier. A 42% reduction in strokes and heart disease, no less, in women taking HRT.[40] No-one seemed particularly concerned that this was an observational study. It was just confirming what everyone knew to be true.

By the early 1990s the benefits of HRT were so widely accepted, that menopausal women were now being actively prescribed it to protect against heart disease and strokes. To do otherwise was considered virtual medical malpractice.

Then along came the HERS study, and the WHI. And it turned out that the 'fact' (female sex hormones protect against heart disease), which was never based on any evidence in the first place, was proven to be untrue. Hold the front page '*Unproven fact disproved*'. Although at the time, these studies caused great shock and upset amongst various opinion leaders. Some flatly refused to accept the findings of the study; some still do.

What really interested me about this saga was *not* that the 'ad-hoc' hypothesis itself was untrue – it was clearly nonsense from the start. No, what really interested me was the broader question. Why are some ideas taken up so quickly, so widely, and with so little questioning, when there is no evidence to support them? And why are other ideas rejected out of hand, even if they are supported?

What are the drivers for this completely unscientific, and essentially emotional, behaviour? As it turns out, people have noted the existence of this phenomenon over the ages.

"When a man finds a conclusion agreeable, he accepts it without argument, but when he finds it disagreeable, he will bring against it all the forces of logic and reason."

Thucydides

More recently a UK surgeon called Wilfred Trotter concluded much the same thing about our inability to accept new ideas.

"The mind likes a strange idea as little as the body likes a strange protein and resists it with similar energy. It would not perhaps be too fanciful to say that a new idea is the most quickly acting antigen known to science."

Wilfred Trotter

Over the years, I have come across more and more examples of 'acceptance without argument', and rapid, 'antigen-like' rejection. At first I thought it was somewhat ironic that medical scientists appear to be the worst at this type of instant acceptance – and dismissal. Are not scientists supposed to be objective seekers of truth? Should they not be willing to go wherever the facts lead them, however inconvenient? Surely scientists should be open-minded?

However, I have come to realise that this is not in the least ironic. In fact, it is probably to be expected. Scientists are just the same as normal mortals – only more so. However, to a far greater extent than most people, scientists become very closely associated with the ideas that they believe in.

In time their reputations and status become inextricably bound up with the hypotheses that they research, and lecture on. Can you imagine the impact of a leading climate change scientist declaring that they had changed their mind, and that man-made global warming is a myth. Just for starters, how do you think they would be treated by their global-warming believing peers? (Not with open arms, I suspect).

The reality is that once a scientist comes to believe that a hypothesis is correct e.g. heart disease is caused by eating saturated fat, which raises cholesterol levels, which causes thickenings in arteries which leads to heart attacks and strokes – the 'diet-heart/cholesterol hypothesis.' Once you believe this, and write articles on it, and gain awards for researching it, and make it your life's work. How easy is it to change?

Very difficult, would be the answer.

"I know that most men, including those at ease with problems of the greatest complexity, can seldom accept even the simplest and most obvious truth, it be such as would oblige them to admit the falsity of conclusions which they have delighted in explaining to colleagues, which they have proudly taught others, and which they have woven, thread by thread, into the fabric of their lives."

Leo Tolstoy

The exceedingly tight connection between what scientists believe, and their sense of worth, and status, explains the angry vehemence with which new ideas are rejected. Indeed, the level of rage that has been directed at me from time to time, has forced me to conclude that when you criticise the ideas of a scientist, you are, effectively, attacking them personally – and they will lash out at you. Their ideas are as jealously protected as if they were their own flesh and blood. In some cases, more so.

The best book on this complex and fascinating subject, and the lengths we are prepared to go to, to protect our ideas, and thus ourselves, is Travis and Aronson's *Mistakes were made (but not by me)*. I recommend everyone in the world to read it. That is, if they want to try to understand themselves a little more, and why they act as they do.

Of course, the flip-side to the rage and anger with which people can react when their ideas are challenged, is the ease with which certain ideas are accepted... *when a man finds a conclusion agreeable he accepts it without argument.* (In order not to be considered sexist, I think women do this too).

At which point, in a slightly roundabout way, I shall return to the female sex hormone hypothesis, and why it was so rapidly, and unquestioningly, accepted. And so, back to heart disease.

Virtually since research began into this area, it had been noticed that women have higher cholesterol levels than men. Despite this, younger women (women aged under about 65), had much lower death rates from heart disease. In most populations it is three to four times less. However the exact proportion varies considerably, from twenty times less (New Zealand in the 1970's), to one and a half times less (Brazil), to zero (black American women).

If you believe that a raised cholesterol level is the most important causal factor for heart disease, then the fact that younger women suffer far few heart attacks, represents a rather inconvenient fact. Shouldn't women actually be at higher risk? It is true that women generally smoke less than men, and this can explain some of the difference.

However, if you plug female and male risk factors into a risk calculator: age, smoking, blood pressure, diabetes, LDL/cholesterol levels, there is still an inexplicable gap. On the face of it, women appear to contradict the cholesterol hypothesis.

When confronted with a possible contradiction, or 'refutation' such as this, you have a number of different choices. You can call it a paradox, you can ignore it, or you can try to explain why it happens. (You could also accept that your hypothesis is wrong... sorry, just a thought).

Calling something a paradox is a method that has been used again and again to explain away many apparent contradictions about heart disease. As a method it explains nothing, but it does have the advantage of placing the issue on the top shelf, far away from prying eyes. 'Oh yes, that, don't worry about it, an explanation will turn up...' However, if no explanation does turn up, at some point you are going to have bring the paradox down from the top shelf, dust it down, and explain it. But calling it a 'paradox' does buy time.

The second choice is to ignore the issue altogether, which is more common than you might think. In this particular case, ignoring the issue takes two forms. The first is to add *'male or female sex'* to the risk factor calculator as a variable. Men are at greater risk than women, so for women you simply divide the male risk by three, or four, or whatever the difference happens to be in your own country.

So you simply re-calculate the risk for women, without ever having to address the issue of *why* it is so different. They have the same risk factors for heart disease, but you have to divide by four to establish their actual risk. Of course this works, in that, it does calculate their risk.

In the same way, in the UK, those from the Asian Subcontinent are at a higher risk of heart disease than the surrounding population – with identical risk factors. Which means that you first calculate their risk, looking at blood pressure, smoking, age etc (all of the established risk factors for heart disease). Then, once you have done this you have to multiply by 1.4.

Changing the risk calculator in this way is all very well, and it does calculate their risk – if you don't think about it too hard. However, as with declaring something to be a paradox, you are always left with the uneasy sense that you have not really solved the problem, merely fudged it. At some point the green shoots of doubt will find the cracks, and emerge once more. *'But why do you have to divide by three, or four, to calculate the risk for women? Why do you have to multiply by 1.4 for Asians?'* Said the ghost of Christmas future. *'Why... why... why...'*

There is also another, rather more complex method of ignoring the issue, which is being increasingly used. This is to use the *lifetime risk* of dying of heart disease. It goes something like this. In the end we are all going to die of something, and a large number of us will die of 'cardiovascular disease (CVD).' As it turns out, in the end, about as many women as men die of cardiovascular disease. Fewer younger women, more older women. So, if you choose to calculate 'lifetime risk of CVD' then there is no major difference between men and women.

Using this method of determining risk, you can state that women are not actually protected by anything. Why... because over a lifetime, they are just as likely as men to die of heart disease. Of course this says nothing about the age at which you will die. Yes, I know. Think about that for too long, and you will almost certainly go mad.

How else can you try to explain away the difference in heart disease between men and women? You could use my preferred explanation, which would be to state that the 'cholesterol hypothesis' is wrong. This certainly works. It also explains the French paradox, the Swiss paradox, the Greek (Crete vs. Corfu) paradox, the Japanese paradox, the Asian paradox, the... (no room for all the paradoxes here).

Sorry, that was a moment of madness. No-one was ever going to use the explanation that actually fits all the facts. Everyone was, and is, far too wedded to the cholesterol hypothesis.

In the end, the best way to explain away the difference in heart disease risk between men and women is to establish a reason why women are 'protected.' And the best place to start is to look for some significant biological difference between the sexes, to see if this may be the cause of the vast chasm in rates of heart disease.

The most obvious biological difference between men and women is their sex hormones. So this seemed a reasonable place to start. Could female sex hormones, via some complex effect (undetermined), explain the vast gap in heart disease rates? Answer... possibly. Well, possibly, seemed to be good enough for most people. And so, with the fair wind of *we really want to believe this'* filling its sails, the good ship *female sex hormone* sailed off.

Given time, lab-based research in rabbits became proof of an effect in humans. The accelerating rate of heart disease after the menopause became further proof – so long as you didn't actually look at the curves properly. Studies on extremely healthy women who took HRT, and developed less heart disease, were grasped hold of gratefully. Gradually, all of this shaky evidence was welded together. 'Possibly' transformed into 'probably'; probably became fact.

The only thing that surprises me about this whole sorry saga is that the HERS study and the WHI study were actually accepted. I thought they would be dismissed as being poorly designed, not using the right dose of hormones, not measuring the right outcomes, etc. etc. This is what normally happens to studies that disprove fondly held hypotheses.

For a while the HERS study, and others in this area, gave me hope that all incorrect scientific dogma can eventually be overturned by the facts. Unfortunately the cholesterol hypothesis still appears completely impervious to such puny weapons as contradictory evidence. Like a monster from a 1950s sci-fi movie, it consumes contradictory evidence and grows ever more powerful.

As a side note, now that the sex hormone hypothesis has gone, what factor *is* thought to protect younger women against heart disease?

Interestingly, this seems to be a question that no-one is much interested in answering any more. It sits on the top shelf, gathering dust. It can't be explained by sex hormones, or cholesterol levels, or any of the traditional risk factors... I suppose it is, you guessed it, a paradox.

Anyway, the more that I have researched heart disease the more I have come to recognise that the sex hormone hypothesis was not some strange anomaly. It was just the first of literally hundreds of unproven 'facts' that are now widely accepted.

Ad-hoc hypotheses

To give you some idea of the scale of this issue. In 1981, the journal *Atherosclerosis* published a list of 246 possible risk factors for heart disease. I have no idea how many there now are – thousands probably. Many sound highly plausible. But when you track them back you realise that the vast majority of them have one thing in common, which makes them instantly suspect. They are what Karl Popper described as ad-hoc hypotheses.

"Ad-hoc hypotheses – that is, at the time untestable auxiliary hypotheses – can save almost any theory from any particular refutation. But this does not mean we can go on with an ad-hoc hypotheses as long as we like. It may become testable; and a negative test may force us either to give it up or to introduce a new secondary ad-hoc hypothesis, and so on, ad infinitum... moreover, the possibility of making things up with ad-hoc hypotheses must not be exaggerated: there are many refutations which cannot be avoided in this way, even though some kind of immunizing tactic such as ignoring the refutation is always possible."

Karl Popper. *The problem of demarcation*

When I first read this, I wasn't quite sure what he was talking about. Surely scientists don't just make things up, then claim they are true. How little I knew. In reality the world of heart disease research has now become jammed solid with *ad-hoc* hypotheses. And more are created on an almost daily basis. Green leaf tea, antioxidants, omega-3 fatty acids, coffee, genetic protection, excess iron, excess copper, or too little copper...

When it comes to the creation of untested auxiliary hypothesis, the French data is the veritable mother lode. This is because the French represent perhaps the greatest single threat to the cholesterol hypothesis. They eat more saturated fat than any other nation in Europe, their cholesterol levels are slightly above average. They smoke more than most, their blood pressure is around average, they don't exercise much, and they have the same BMI as most other countries. Yet, despite all of this, they have the lowest rate of heart disease in Europe. One-third the rate in the USA, and UK (women and men under 65) – and still falling.

What possible explanation, or explanations, can be there be for this fact? The first immunising tactic used was to call it a paradox. In fact it was described exactly this way in many prestigious journals, from the *NEJM* to the *The Lancet* and the *BMJ*. (And still is).

However, as mentioned before, you can't really keep on calling something a paradox forever. Especially when you are talking about a country with 60 million people in it. This is not just one paradox... mais non. It represents 60 million living, breathing paradoxes. Therefore, in the end you must try to explain what 'protects' them. Here is a short selection of the ad-hoc hypothesis developed:

- The French incorrectly certify deaths from heart disease i.e. they don't really have a low rate of heart disease – proven wrong by the WHO MONICA study (but still widely believed, and often quoted as gospel).

- Red wine protects against heart disease – no outcome evidence.

- Garlic protects against heart disease – no evidence at all.

- Lightly cooked vegetables, which retain antioxidants, protect against heart disease – no evidence.

- The French have not had a high intake of saturated fat for long enough for it to affect their heart disease rate. The 'time-lag' hypothesis. If we wait, this hypothesis suggests, we will see their rate accelerate. This top level gibberish was proposed in 1998. Fourteen years later the French rate of heart disease was still falling rapidly. Oops, bong. Please strike this hypothesis from the record... fat chance.

I have looked into these ad-hoc hypotheses and many, many, many more. In the final analysis, they all have four things in common.

One, they were developed with one purpose in mind – to immunize against refutations to the cholesterol hypothesis. Two, they very rapidly become very widely accepted throughout the scientific community. Three, they have no clinical outcome data to support them. Four... they are not true.

In fact, now that I more fully understand what is actually going on, it has made it relatively simple for me to gauge the truth, or otherwise, of the new 'risk factors' for heart disease that are announced almost every day.

Just to pick a recent one at random that you may have heard of. "Chemicals found within chocolate protects against heart disease."

I read this headline and I thought... Well you don't really need to know what my first thought was. However, in order to decide if this were likely to be true I asked myself the question. Is this an ad-hoc hypothesis? If so, treat as highly unlikely.

So I took a few steps backwards. According to the diet-heart/cholesterol hypothesis, chocolate is high in fat, and fat raises cholesterol levels. So, chocolate should cause heart disease, should it not? In fact, chocolate consumption has been found to be associated with a reduction in the risk of heart disease. This contradicts the cholesterol hypothesis, and so an ad-hoc hypothesis was required to fill this hole.

Now, if I were trying to protect the cholesterol hypothesis, what would I do? I would find some chemical in chocolate – there are many. Then I would do a study to demonstrate that one or more of these chemicals had some physiological effect to explain chocolate's protective effects.

Lo and behold, researchers in Sweden (and Swedish researchers always seem the most believable, somehow), have found that catechins and procyanidines, found in dark chocolate, inhibit the enzyme Angiotensin Converting Enzyme (ACE).[41] When ACE is blocked, blood pressure drops. Indeed, this is actually how the class of drugs known as ACE-inhibitors (Blood Pressure (BP) lowering drugs) work.

Things became even more promising when researchers found that healthy volunteers given dark chocolate demonstrated an 18% reduction in ACE activity. This is comparable to the effect seen with ACE-inhibitors. It was all looking good, and a story was being stitched together. Hold the front page. We have a biological plausible explanation, and real scientific data to support it.

But before you get too carried away, and start believing headlines such as 'Why chocolate protects against heart disease,' you should step back and ask yourself. What is missing here? Apart from a five-year-long double-blind, randomised controlled study, obviously.

What is missing here is a clinical effect. Something mentioned almost in passing by the authors was that there was no drop in blood pressure in those taking cocoa extract. They stated that this actually meant nothing. In fact the lack of impact on blood pressure was '*exactly as expected*', as it would require a longer time period than the 18 days of the study to see any impact on blood pressure reduction.

Does this sound reasonable? Well, it does, on first hearing. Ad-hoc explanations piled on top of ad-hoc hypotheses always appear superficially reasonable. But is it likely to be true? Could it really take more than 18 days for a de-facto ACE-inhibitor to lower blood pressure?

To find out, I decided to review the Cochrane collaboration meta-analysis of all ACE-inhibitor studies to find out how long it takes a pharmaceutical ACE-inhibitor to lower blood pressure. The answer is, between 1 and 12 hours. '*ACE inhibitors reduced BP measured 1 to 12 hours after the dose.*'[42] To be frank, I already had my doubts about the author's explanation as to why BP did not drop. For the simple reason that one of the widely recognised problems of ACE-inhibitors is that they very rapidly lower blood pressure. So much so, indeed, that you have to start with a very low dose, and gradually increase it to ensure that serious hypotension does not occur. At one time ACE-inhibitors were only dispensed in hospital to avoid this problem. Now they are handed out like Smarties in GP surgeries.

In short, it is widely known – and proven beyond any shadow of doubt – that ACE-inhibitors reduce blood pressure rapidly. Yet, when you eat cocoa extract, which allegedly reduces ACE activity by as much as an ACE-inhibitor, there is no drop in blood pressure – even after 18 days. And if the blood pressure doesn't drop, how does dark chocolate provide any benefits? Through the power of dark chocolateyness, no doubt.

Once again, as with all ad-hoc hypotheses, we have an idea that sounds highly plausible... if you don't look too closely. But if you dig down deeper, there is a well-camouflaged, but fatal flaw in the evidence. This is far from unusual. In fact, a vital missing link is a common feature of almost all ad-hoc hypotheses. They are like conjuring tricks for the mind. You think you have been told everything to provide a plausible explanation, but the clinical evidence card has been cunningly hidden up the researcher's sleeve.

This does not mean that chocolate does not protect against heart disease through some chemical effect. It may do, it may not. But up to this point, the research has proven nothing. It may be that eating chocolate is so enjoyable that it releases chemicals in the brain that protect you from heart disease. Or it may be that enjoying yourself is good for your health (my preferred explanation).

Equally some ad-hoc hypotheses might be true. Omega 3 fatty acids do reduce the death rate from heart disease (they have an antiarrhythmic effect, which helps to prevent sudden cardiac death, and this has been proven in long-term controlled outcome studies). Also smoking, which was never part of the diet-heart hypothesis does cause – or at least accelerate – heart disease. Just because a hypothesis is an ad-hoc hypothesis does not inevitably mean it is wrong.

But the vast majority of these ad-hoc hypotheses are wrong. Just to touch on one final, example, mentioned earlier on. Red wine protects against heart disease. Most people believe this is true. Indeed, if you type the words 'red *wine heart disease'* into *PubMed* you will be deluged with 'evidence' of its protective effects. You will also be inundated with chemical names, such as: resveratrol, and polyphenols and procyanidines, (you may recognise them from the cocoa story) and antioxidants. All of which have 'proven' effects on heart disease.

It will all seem very reasonable, and plausible, and believable, and thousands of papers have been written on this exact topic. You can even buy bottles of wine based on their protective effect on heart disease, dependent on the concentration of resveratrol. Thud! (Head hits desk once more).

But if you decide to look for the outcome study demonstrating that red wine reduces the risk of heart disease you will look long and hard. And I can guarantee that you find nothing. Yes, the French drink red wine and have a low rate of heart disease. This is not proof of anything. Rich middle class people in the US also drink red wine, and they too have lower rates of heart disease than the surrounding population... quelle surprise. (See under HRT).

But the main reason why I can be virtually certain that red wine does not protect against heart disease (any more than moderate consumption of any other form of alcohol) is because of why the idea was born. As an ad-hoc hypothesis designed to protect the cholesterol hypothesis from a refutation by the French. Pure and simple.

At this point I think I may have illustrated that things that are not true are commonly held to be true. You will hopefully also have seen the main reason for this – we become invested in a belief and when something undermines that belief we will find something else to prop up our original belief. There need be no end to the number of ad-hoc hypotheses created to address no end of paradoxes. These are no more true than the original untruth, but they will be commonly held to be so.

Footnote:

Whilst writing this section, a small news story appeared about resveratrol.

"A University of Connecticut researcher known for touting the health benefits of red wine is guilty of 145 counts of fabricating and falsifying data with image-editing software, according to a 3-year university investigation made public Wednesday."[43]

Yes, here is another problem with medical research. Some of it (I have no idea how much), is just plain made up.

CHAPTER FIVE

Reducing numbers does not equal reducing risk

When I started to write about how data are manipulated, why, and by whom, I thought I would be finished after about 20 pages. There could not possibly be much more to write than this, I thought.

However, when I try to explain things, I realise that the issues go down deeper and deeper, with far more issues being interconnected at all levels. For instance, when I look at an area such as blood-pressure lowering and I see a statement about benefits, I know that they will be using the log-linear model and surrogate end-points.

Then I think, how best to explain this to an intelligent and interested audience. First, what the heck is a log-linear model? Then, what is a surrogate end-point? Where do these things come from and what do they mean, and why do they matter at all? What seems very clear in my mind, after 30 years of living with this nonsense, ends up needing a great deal of explanation.

Surrogate end-points

Let's start with surrogate end-points and we'll use blood pressure to help with our explanation. A surrogate end-point is a measure that substitutes for an actual clinical event. You will be very familiar with this term if you live in my 'Alice in Wonderland' cholesterol world. The European register on nutrition and health claims allows the following claim to be put on stuff containing plant sterols: "*Plant sterols and plant stanol esters have been shown to lower/reduce blood cholesterol.*"[44]

The surrogate end-point in this case is lowering the cholesterol measurement. It has become one of those "things that are not true,

91

commonly held to be true", that lowering cholesterol is a good thing all by itself. It is so obviously beneficial that we do not need to demonstrate any actual clinical benefit (e.g. fewer people died). That's one surrogate end-point for you.

Moving on to blood pressure. It has been known for many years that a high blood pressure is associated with a higher risk of heart attacks, and strokes… and many other things e.g. kidney damage, aortic aneurysms, heart failure and suchlike. (For the sake of reasonable simplicity, I am only going to focus on heart attacks and stroke here). Please also note the use of the word '*associated*' from the outset.

It has also become widely accepted that the risk of raised blood pressure is continuous, with no upper and lower range. In addition, almost everyone agrees that the danger accelerates as the pressure rises higher. This is known as 'logarithmic' increase in risk along a straight line base, and it is why the model is sometimes referred to as 'log-linear'. For the sake of simplicity, I shall only refer to this as the linear model.

This simple paradigm guides all thinking in this area, and the underlying concept was most famously coined by Jeremiah Stamler in 1991.

"The relation of SBP [systolic blood pressure] to risk of death is continuous, graded, and strong, and there is no evidence of a threshold."[45]

In simple graphical form the relationship between blood pressure and cardiovascular risk looks something like the graph below. I created this by inputting figures from the latest cardiovascular disease prevention guidelines, published in the US in 2013.

As the blood pressure rises, the risk of a cardiovascular 'event' (heart attack, or stoke) also rises. At higher pressures the curve does start to accelerate upwards. (Although I must admit that it is not very clear from this particular graph).

You may wonder what happens at a systolic blood pressure below 90 mmHg? Well, you cannot input figures below this level, as the model does not accept them. Why not? That is probably a discussion for another day. (Something to do with the fact that 'hypotension', otherwise known as dangerously low blood pressure, starts at a systolic BP of 90 mmHg).

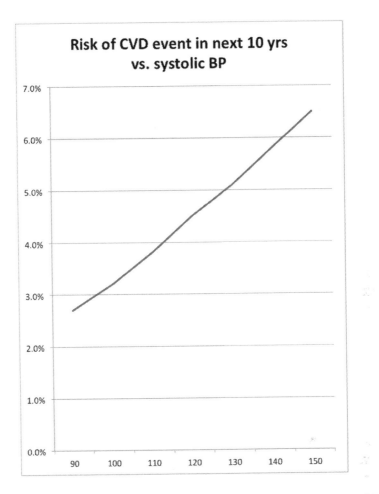

Risk of CVD event in next 10 yrs vs. systolic BP

So unquestioned is the belief in this model that you can use blood pressure as a 'surrogate' end-point for true clinical benefit. By which I mean that if you lower blood pressure by 10 mmHg, by whatever technique you choose, you do not need to do a five-year long clinical trial to see if heart attacks and strokes are actually prevented.

All you need to do is to use the model to calculate the benefit that would inevitably accrue. Lowering blood pressure is, thus, a 'surrogate' end-point. Pressure lowered, benefit achieved... check.

Pharmaceutical companies love surrogate end-points; primarily because these end-points save the companies vast amounts of time and money.

If you are required to set up a clinical study to demonstrate that your drug actually has some outcome benefit, this can take many years. You may also need to recruit thousands of patients, sometimes tens of thousands. This is because it usually takes a very large number of people a long time for enough of them to die during your study period to show any statistically significant difference in mortality.

On the other hand, if all you have to do is demonstrate that you can reduce the blood pressure by 10 mmHg to achieve a mortality benefit, you need far fewer participants. Also, the study may only need to last months, even weeks, before you have enough data to launch your drug.

The increased value of this to the industry can be measured in tens of billions of dollars. Maybe hundreds of billions. Perhaps, if you added together all the drugs launched on the back of surrogate end-points over the years... Trillions.

Not only do you save hundreds of millions by not having to run massive studies, your drug can make money for far longer. The patent on drugs lasts 22 years, from the initial registration of the compound. That is when the clock starts ticking.

If you get rid of the need for lengthy clinical trials, you can shave five years off the drug development time. That represents five more years where your drug faces no competition, anywhere in the world. Assuming a 'blockbuster' drug can make five billion per year, five years of extra patent protection is worth twenty five billion in additional dosh.

Surrogate end-points are not confined to blood-pressure lowering, far from it. From our cholesterol explanation of surrogate end-points, did you know that atorvastatin, which is the best-selling statin of all time, was launched with no outcome data? Yet it became the most widely prescribed drug in the history of medicine purely on the basis that it lowered cholesterol, and must therefore prevent heart attacks and strokes.

For many years Pfizer were forced to include this little snippet at the bottom of their adverts in the US: *"Lipitor has not been shown to prevent heart disease or heart attacks."*[46]

I would be willing to bet that you did not know that.

But boy did Lipitor lower cholesterol; and boy did it make money. Tens of billions per year, until the patent ran out. This is perhaps the most powerful single example why surrogate end-points are enormously valuable to the industry. In this case, around $125 billion in sales, for one drug.[47]

However, whilst surrogate end-points are enormously profitable, and thus popular, if they are misused they can also be rather disastrous. For many years two drugs, encainide and flecainide were widely used to suppress cardiac arrhythmias. Cardiac arrhythmias can be fatal, and it was assumed that suppression of these potentially fatal arrhythmias would save many lives.

It is true that encainide and flecainide[vi] are very good at suppressing arrhythmias on an Electro Cardio Gram (ECG). Essentially, a surrogate end-point. Indeed, entirely on the basis of their ability to 'cure' ECGs they were very widely prescribed. Mainly in the US. As it turns out, they were also rather effective at killing people.

When an outcome study was eventually done (CAST), it had to be stopped prematurely because it became obvious that the two drugs were wiping people out.[48] Thomas Moore, a scientist who has worked in drug safety and policy for 20 years, estimated that these drugs killed over 60,000 people.[49] Not bad going, not bad at all. More than the total number of American soldiers who died in the Vietnam War.[50] *Pharmaceutical products – far more effective at killing people than the Viet Cong.'*

More recently, but somewhat less apocalyptically, we have ezetimibe. This drug lowers cholesterol, but through a very different mechanism than statins. Because it lowered cholesterol, ezetimibe was not required to show any impact on heart disease and strokes. It was launched purely on the basis of its cholesterol lowering ability. It has since made billions upon billions.

As you may have guessed, when a study was finally done to look at its effect on heart attacks and strokes, it was found that ezetimibe was completely and utterly useless. As expected this did not have the slightest effect on the prescribing on ezetimibe. Nor has it led to any real questioning of the use of cholesterol lowering as a surrogate end-point.

Another example of where altering a surrogate end-point caused harm, rather than benefit, is in the area of weight gain in pregnancy. It was known that increased weight gain resulted in raised blood pressure and eclampsia (dangerously high blood pressure) with far worse fetal outcomes.

On this basis, women were advised to keep weight gain in pregnancy to under twenty pounds. When women did manage to control weight gain (a surrogate end-point) there was a reduction in both the rate of hypertension and eclampsia. However, as pointed out in this paper in *Hypertension*:

---

vi Flecainide is now used, very effectively, to treat certain forms of heart arrhythmias. The problem with flecainde was using it in far too wide a set of indications where any benefits were overwhelmed by harm.

95

"...medical interventions must be tested for their effects on human health, in addition to determining whether the intervention will be able to produce the targeted effect. For example, in an analogous situation, pregnant women were once advised to limit weight gain during pregnancy to <20 pounds to reduce the risk of rising blood pressure and eclampsia. In fact, this did produce those two desired outcomes. Unfortunately, and unexpectedly, limiting weight gain in pregnancy increased fetal morbidity and mortality rates. Women are no longer advised to limit weight gain in pregnancy."[51]

All of this should make it very clear that, just because risk goes up when a measurement goes up, this does not mean we are looking at a cause. Even if it is a cause, lowering the 'measurement' may still do more harm than good, for reasons that you may not have initially predicted.

As a simple example of unexpected harm, we know that lowering the blood pressure does reduce the risk of stroke. However, taking blood-pressure lowering drugs also makes it more likely that you will fall because your blood pressure drops when you try to stand (postural hypotension). A particular problem for the elderly. A fall can result in a fractured hip, and the operation to repair the hip could well kill you. End result, more harm than good.

"People over 70 years old who are taking drugs for high blood pressure seem to be at a higher risk of fall injury, such as hip fracture or head injury, than those who are not being treated, especially if they have had a previous fall, a study has found."[52]

Another area where intensive lowering of a surrogate end-point backfired was with the ACCORD study. Over 10,000 people were enrolled. Half of those in the study were supposed to get blood sugar down a moderate amount; the other half went into an intensive treatment arm. In the intensive treatment arm all possible medications were used to drive blood glucose down as much as possible. The conclusions of the study were, as follows: *"Intensive glucose lowering increased the risk of cardiovascular disease and total mortality in younger participants..."*[53]

There was a 71% relative increase risk (RR) of early death in those under the age of 65. This trial was halted early due to the greatly increased risk of death in those receiving intensive treatment. So, high sugar levels are bad, but if you try to get them down too far, you increased mortality by 71% RR. Why? All sorts of reasons I would imagine.

Closely related to this is the example of the drug Avandia. It was assumed that this drug would be highly beneficial for diabetics, because it helped control blood sugar. Diabetes is associated with a three to five fold risk in heart attack death, and Avandia lowers blood sugar levels.

However, a study published in the *New England Journal of Medicine* found that Avandia increased the risk of heart attack by 43% and increased the risk of death from cardiovascular causes by 64%. These data have been questioned, but only after intense lobbying from GSK. The drug has been reinstated in the US, but remains banned in Europe.[54]

Blood pressure

I could give many more such examples of numbers being lowered without risk being lowered. A surrogate end-point being 'improved' with an apparently paradoxical increase in death rates, but I am going to focus on blood pressure medication to look at why a surrogate end-point may be a far more complex beast than it seems.

The other reason is that more people take blood-pressure lowering tablets than any other type of drug. Almost everyone knows their blood pressure, and doctors and nurses measure it constantly. Surely this is one area where the benefit of lowering has been proven beyond doubt. It must be true that lowering blood pressure is highly beneficial... mustn't it? This is not just any old surrogate end-point.

Well maybe; maybe not. Or maybe just... not. To my mind there are four issues with treating blood pressure, which have not really been resolved:

1. What is raised blood pressure? (Is it a disease?)

2. What are we treating when we lower blood pressure?

3. Can we really believe in the linear model?

4. How can we interpret the results? (Blood-pressure lowering tablets have many different effects, which make interpreting the results from the clinical trials almost impossible).

1. What is raised blood pressure?

The first problem in this area starts when you try to analyse what a raised blood pressure might be in the first place. What is it and what causes it? Do we really understand it? In a small number of people a 'cause' can be found. Around 10% of cases would fit into this category. Obviously, here, a raised blood pressure is clearly a symptom of an underlying disease.

When a cause can be found, the blood pressure can normally be brought down by treating the underlying condition. However, in the vast majority of cases no reasons can be found. This is when we call raised blood pressure – *essential hypertension*. This translates back into English as *'raised blood pressure of unknown cause.'*

It must be said that calling it essential hypertension does sound a bit more scientific and professional. It is better than wringing your hands in despair and admitting to the patient that *'Your blood pressure is high, and I haven't the slightest damned idea why. I'm sorry. Yes, I am utterly useless, am I not?'* Sob.

Rather than put doctors into this vulnerable position, it came to pass that an admission of defeat became a disease. *'I must inform you that, after running many, many tests, I have been able to diagnose your condition. You have essential hypertension.'*

'Thank goodness you managed to diagnose it doctor, now what can you do about it?'

For many years there was nothing much that could be done. A few patients with very, very high blood pressure known as 'malignant hypertension' had a part of their nervous system severed. An operation known as a sympathectomy. (An operation which is seeing a return of sorts).

This was done because the sympathetic nervous system drives the kidneys to produce various hormones that raise blood pressure. This system also constricts the arteries, and increases the heart rate and suchlike, which further raises the blood pressure.

This all happens because the sympathetic nervous system is a key player in the 'fight or flight' response. When activated it revs up your entire physiology to either fight, or run away. So it is no surprise that when the sympathetic nervous system is activated it has major effects on the blood pressure. If you sever the sympathetic nerves, the blood pressure must fall.

Another tactic was to cut salt intake to, virtually, zero using the Kempner diet. This diet was, completely tasteless, unappetizing, and insipid. Very few patients could tolerate it for any length of time. It consisted of boiled or steamed rice in plain water with no salt, and very little fruit (except dates, avocados, and dried or canned fruit).

Water and fluids were also restricted. Even among the very few who could tolerate this diet, the reductions in blood pressure were pretty small, and probably did not exceed the random spontaneous variations in blood pressure. In short it did not actually work.

Then came the drugs.

Shortly after the drugs came the clinical trials. Now there is no doubt that when the blood pressure is exceedingly high, lowering the pressure is beneficial. The first two trials on BP lowering were very positive... amazingly positive. In the US Veterans Study, 27 out of 70 untreated hypertensive patients sustained strokes, with only 2 out of 70 in the treated group. This is a 1,350% absolute risk difference.

I have to tell you that I harbour my doubts about this study. Yes, blood pressure does increase the risk of a stroke. However, a rate of stroke of nearly one in two (27/70), in a single year, is almost unbelievably high. So almost unbelievably high that I might even struggle to believe it. But believe it I shall learn to do.

Leaving aside my doubts about such studies, and assuming them to be completely accurate, means that I am not discussing catastrophically high blood pressure here. The sort of level that might affect 1 in 1,000 people. I am discussing blood pressure that is somewhat raised. Mild to moderate hypertension, if those terms mean anything anymore. They did at one time, but this is a world of ever moving targets and nomenclature. A veritable tower of Babel.

Despite the difficulty of ever pinning anything down when it comes to terminology in this area, I will use the term 'mild hypertension'. This covers the vast majority of people who have a raised blood pressure. At the risk of being immediately shot down I shall use the upper figures of 160 systolic and 110 diastolic as the upper range.[vii]

Having just said that, for the sake of further simplicity I am only going to look at systolic blood pressure. It may not be absolutely perfect to do so, but getting into the value of systolic vs. diastolic BP measurement and the lowering thereof would fill several books. They would be exceedingly boring books, but people seem to become enormously aerated about such things.

At this point I feel that I do need to take a step back and reiterate the fact that as the blood pressure goes up, the risk of heart attack and stroke also goes up. I don't think anyone would disagree with that statement. However, and here we hit the first point of conflict, this does *not* mean that high blood pressure causes heart attacks and strokes.

---

vii Systolic pressure represents the maximum blood pressure in the system, just after the heart has contracted. Diastolic represents the lowest pressure, just before the heart contracts again. The pressure never drops to zero, or anywhere near.

We could be looking at the equivalent of yellow fingers and smoking. By which I mean that the disease leading to heart attacks and strokes could also cause the blood pressure to be high. Therefore, lowering the blood pressure may be as useless as scrubbing your fingers clean to prevent lung cancer.

An even more radical thought is that heart disease, and stroke risk, could be the underlying disease(s) leading to high blood pressure; not the other way around. By which I mean that the causal chain is not:

Raised blood pressure → increased risk of heart attack and stroke

Instead it is:

Heart disease and '*stroke disease*' → raised blood pressure

To some people this will be immediately intuitive. For others, bear with me for a page or two whilst I run through a thought experiment for you. It starts with two examples:

If you have a narrowed artery leading to one or both of your kidneys, your blood pressure will be extremely high. This is because the kidneys are the key organs that monitor and control blood pressure. Reduction of blood flow to the kidneys activates the renin-angiotensin system, which will sharply raise blood pressure, thus restoring 'normal' blood supply to the kidneys.

In this situation if you open up the narrowed renal artery and restore normal blood flow, the kidney stops producing hormones that raise the blood pressure and the pressure drops. In this case the narrowed blood vessel is clearly and unequivocally the cause of raised blood pressure.

Another example where narrowed arteries raise the blood pressure is when blood clots build up in the lungs. This can happen for various reasons, but it is almost always a result of repeated deep vein thrombosis (DVTs). These break off and travel into the lungs where they get stuck causing a pulmonary embolism (PE).

Assuming the PEs do not kill you – which they often do – the build-up of these blood clots increases the resistance to blood flow through the lungs. This requires the right side of the heart to pump harder and harder to force the blood through the obstructed blood vessels. (The right side of the heart pumps the blood into the lungs before the blood returns to the left side of the heart, which pumps it round the rest of the body. Arteries in the lungs are therefore called veins, and vice-versa).

This leads to a condition known as pulmonary hypertension (raised blood pressure in the lungs). At first the heart can pump harder and harder by building up the heart muscle in the right side (right ventricular hypertrophy). Eventually, however, the heart has to work too hard and starts to pack in. A condition known as right heart failure.

There is one way to cure this condition. You can do an operation to pull all of the clots out of the lung. This is called a *'pulmonary thromboendarterectomy.'* Normally, all the clots have joined together to form a mould of the vascular tree which can be yanked out in one go. As you can probably imagine, removing a large mass of clot from the lungs is a dangerous procedure with a high mortality rate.

However, if the operation is a success, the blood pressure in the lungs returns to normal, and the right side of the heart also returns to normal. Remove the resistance, and all of the downstream problems simply disappear. Including the raised blood pressure.

If we turn this discussion back to the rest of circulatory system, we know that the main underlying problem in both heart disease and stroke is that the arteries become narrowed by atherosclerotic plaques.

Which means that here is a new model for you to think about:

- Heart disease and stroke are, basically, conditions of narrowed and thickened arteries;

- Narrowed and thickened arteries reduce blood flow to various critical organs;

- Reduced blood flow triggers the kidneys to raise the blood pressure;

- The blood pressure goes up creating 'essential hypertension';

- The left ventricle has to pump harder to maintain flow;

- Left ventricular hypertrophy develops, then heart failure.

What is wrong with this model? I shall let you think about it, and try to find a flaw.

There are, however, a couple of problems with demonstrating this model to be correct. First, measuring the total resistance of the arterial system is tricky – if not impossible. Secondly, unlike with pulmonary emboli in the lungs, you cannot reach into the body and pull our great plugs of blood clot, thus returning the blood pressure to normal. Clots like this do not exist in arteries around the body. Or, if they do, it is usually a pretty accurate clinical sign that you are, in fact, dead.

Anyway, at this point I hope you can see why it is not actually madness to claim that cardiovascular disease (CVD) may be the cause of high blood pressure rather than the other way round. Another strong argument in favour of this model is that it actually makes sense, whereas the current universally accepted model does not.

To believe that essential hypertension is a disease requires you to accept that the blood pressure rises for no reason, then it goes on to cause damage around the body. Personally I am not keen on the idea that we can create diseases 'de facto' by giving a medical symptom a fancy Latin name 'essential hypertension'. At which point we do not need to look for a cause. Res Ipsa Loquitur (the thing speaks for itself), as the Latins used to say.

All of this raises the question, when we lower the blood pressure what are we actually doing? Treating a disease, or a symptom of a disease? And if we are treating a symptom, how likely is it that we are going be curing the underlying disease? Discuss.

2. What are we 'treating' when we lower blood pressure?

Another more direct problem with the current model of blood-pressure lowering is as follows. With heart attacks and stroke we actually have three completely distinct mechanisms going on, leading to three different terminal events.

Starting with heart attacks. The mechanism leading to a heart attack is almost universally a blockage of a coronary artery due to thrombus (blood clot). This normally happens at an area of narrowing in an artery supplying blood to the heart (coronary artery). Sudden formation of a thrombus often occurs due to 'rupture' of the narrowing (atherosclerotic plaque) itself. This releases a variety of substances that stimulate a clot to form right on top of the ruptured area, thus completely blocking the artery.

With a stroke there are two very different mechanisms that can occur. In the first, a thrombus breaks off from an area of atherosclerosis in an artery in the neck. The clot then travels up into the brain, and, when the artery narrows, the clot gets stuck. This blocks the blood supply to an area of the brain, and you will suffer an ischaemic stroke. (Ischaemia means lack of blood supply). This is similar to a heart attack.

There is however, a completely different form of stroke, a haemorrhagic stroke. This is where a weakened artery in the brain bursts – usually due to high blood pressure. This causes a bleed into the brain, known as a haemorrhagic stroke.

The important point here is that the two types of stroke are clinically indistinguishable, and are very often clumped together in medical statistics as 'stroke.' But whilst the signs and symptoms are identical, the underlying disease process is completely different. It would surely be remarkable if both types of stroke could be prevented by the same thing – lowering the blood pressure.

Would it not be more likely that a haemorrhagic (bleeding) stroke would be caused by a raised blood pressure; and could be prevented by lowering the pressure? Equally, would it not be far less likely that lowering the blood pressure would not have much, if any, effect on thrombi forming, or breaking off from atherosclerotic plaques in the neck. Nor would there be much, if any, effect on plaque rupture in a coronary artery – causing a heart attack.

Yet, we are supposed to believe that lowering the blood pressure benefits heart attacks and both types of stroke by very nearly the same amount.

The reality is that the results of the blood-pressure lowering trials would give lie to the current model. Indeed, they appear to fully support the 'three mechanism' model of heart disease and strokes. Here, once again, are the results from the original MRC study on lowering blood pressure.

	BP lowering medication	Placebo
Fatal strokes	18	27
Fatal Coronary events (MIs)	106	97
Stroke + (MI) deaths	124	124
Deaths	248	253

As you can see, there were nine fewer stroke deaths, and nine more heart attack deaths. I suspect the reduction in stroke deaths was entirely due to haemorrhagic stroke, but there is no way of knowing this for sure. Why did the rate of heart disease deaths go up? I do not know. Maybe lowering the blood pressure has independently damaging effects on the heart. Maybe it was another direct action of the drugs themselves.

However, the main point here is that the death rates went pretty much in the way expected once you understand the underlying mechanism of strokes and heart attacks. Strokes down, heart disease up a bit.

As a slight aside, I feel I should mention that the MRC study on mild hypertension was the silent earthquake that alerted me to the fact that medical research was not exactly the dispassionate search for truth that I had hoped. Like most people, and almost all doctors, I just believed what the 'experts' said.

I have long since learned my lesson.

3. Can we really believe in the linear model?

Due to my Damascene conversion, I have tended to view all of the evidence about blood-pressure lowering through a filter set to '*maximum skepticism*'. Which means that for the last 20 years or so I have tended to look out for the studies and articles that contradict the linear model of blood pressure, rather than those that support it.

Such articles appear on a reasonably regular basis. They are ignored with precisely the same regularity. My all-time favourite study comes from the year 2000, and it was published in the *European Heart Journal*. It was entitled "There is a non-linear relationship between mortality and blood pressure." It was written by two statisticians and a cardiologist from the University of California, Los Angeles.[55]

What they first did was to go back to the data from the Framingham study (this is the longest ever population study, which has been going on in the town of Framingham in Massachusetts since 1948) and re-analyse it. The reason for this is that the Framingham data laid the foundations for the linear model. In fact the entire edifice of blood-pressure lowering sits on top of the Framingham data. So if these data are wrong then...

These researchers noted that Ancel Keys, yes him, had analysed the Framingham data 20 years before them and used a simple graphical model to review the raw figures themselves. His conclusion was that *"the linear model, in terms of the relationship of overall and coronary heart disease death to blood pressure was unjustified."*

The researchers in 2000 went a great deal further than that. They stated:

"Shockingly, we have found that the Framingham data in no way supported the current paradigm to which they gave birth. In fact, these data actually statistically rejected the linear model. This fact has major consequences. Statistical theory now tells us that paradigm MUST be false..."

104

Amazingly, at least it would have amazed me 20 years ago, the Framingham data completely contradict the linear model. In fact, the lack of association is so clear cut that two statisticians stated that it MUST be false. Their use of capital letters, not mine. Bold words from statisticians, not normally noted for hyperbole.

Has this paper ever been refuted? No, it has not. Sadly, it was given the worst possible treatment that can be dished out by the medical establishment. It was completely ignored. These researchers didn't get anywhere near stage two... vicious personal attacks. Clearly, they were not even considered worthy of crushing.

However, more pertinent to this discussion, this group of researchers went on to say:

"No randomised trial has ever demonstrated any reduction of the risk of either overall or cardiovascular death by reducing systolic blood pressure from our thresholds to below 140 mmHg... It is widely believed that randomized studies have proved that lowering blood pressure is beneficial. Actually, that is not true..."

So, there you have it, according to their meticulous analysis, lowering mildly raised blood pressure does not do any good either. I suppose you may be thinking that this paper is now rather old. There must be other studies since then that have refuted it. Dr Kendrick is just picking papers to suit his argument.

To which I would say, have you not been paying attention at the back. The benefits of blood-pressure lowering, whatever the level, became so widely accepted years ago that it has not been possible, ethically,[viii] to do a placebo-controlled study for a long time. I am not aware of any placebo-controlled trials that have been done in the last twenty years, or so.

This means the only 'new' studies done are to use one type of drug vs. another, or one drug vs. two, or three. Or different combinations in different medical conditions.

Occasionally, if you look very carefully, you can spot groups of patients taking nothing at all to lower their raised blood pressure. For example, here is a very big one called "Association Between Cardiovascular Outcomes and Antihypertensive Drug Treatment in Older Women."[56]

---

viii Not to prescribe a blood-pressure lowering drug to someone with high blood pressure is considered medical malpractice. Therefore, any study with a placebo arm would be rejected by any 'ethics' committee.

This study looked at 93,676 women over a period of 6 years, which is the largest study I have seen in this area. It was essentially designed to look at women taking different types of drugs; either as monotherapy (one bit of 'therapy') or in various combinations. It was not a randomised placebo-controlled study, but an observational study.

However, it was so large that the results are worthy of consideration. I am not going to dissect this study in great detail, although I had to read it very, very carefully to find the nuggets that I was looking for. The first of these nuggets was the following: *"Monotherapy with diuretics was equal or superior to other monotherapy in preventing CVD complications of high blood pressure."*

In short, diuretics were as good, if not better, than any other form of blood-pressure lowering medication. You may remember that diuretics were one of the drugs used in the MRC study, all those years ago. Which means that you are not going to get anything better than the results of the MRC study, even with the newer and far more expensive drugs.

The second nugget was far more difficult to find, as it was not in the abstract, introduction or discussion, and only mentioned in passing.

"We did compare those receiving no medications with those receiving diuretics as mono- therapy and found the HRs[ix] and 95% CIs[x] for coronary disease, stroke, and CVD death to be, respectively, 0.87 (0.72-1.05), 1.05 (0.77-1.41), and 0.92 (0.63-1.33). The baseline systolic BP of the no medications group was higher (149 mmHg) than for those receiving drug treatment."

As usual bland, bland, words. But the findings were quite stunning. The 18,969 women with hypertension who were taking medication, were *more* likely to die from cardiovascular disease during the six year follow-up than those taking *no* medication at all – even though their blood pressure was far higher.

This was true in seven out of the eight drug groups. This was also true, even though the average systolic pressure of the women taking blood-pressure lowering drugs was 8-16 mmHg lower than the women taking no blood pressure drugs.

---

ix   A Hazard Ratio (HR) of 1.0 = average risk. HR 1.2 = 20% increase in risk.

x   A Confidence Interval (CI) of 95% captures the range into which 95% of results fall. If the CI includes 1.0, this is described as not statistically significant.

Just to tease out the results and make them a little clearer. In those women with high blood pressure who were *not* taking any medication the results were:

Heart disease	= 13% lower (non-significant)
Stroke	= 5% higher (non-significant)
Overall CV death	= 8% lower (non-significant)

You may think you can dismiss these results because they were not statistically significant. However, they do significantly fail to disprove the null hypothesis. The null hypothesis being that drug treatment is better than placebo. (You who shall live by statistics shall also die by statistics).

Another thing that fascinates me here, harking back to my earlier point, is that those taking diuretics were less likely to suffer a stroke, and more likely to have a heart attack. This is *exactly* same the pattern as seen in the original MRC study. Which strongly suggests that this was no chance finding.

And what, gentle reader, can we learn from all this?

First, that it is damned hard work finding the information that you are looking for with regard to blood-pressure lowering, but you can find it if you look hard enough. Secondly, that blood-pressure lowering may not be as super-wonderfully brilliant as you may have been led to believe. At least not in the mildly hypertensive range.

Finally, it must be pretty clear by now that the linear model is the most complete nonsense. If women with higher blood pressure are observed to do better than those whose blood pressure was lowered with drugs, then we do not need fancy statistical tests to tell us that Stamler's bold assertion:

"The relation of SBP [systolic blood pressure] to risk of death is continuous, graded, and strong, and there is no evidence of a threshold."

... is completely and utterly wrong.

4. How can we interpret the results?

Despite what you may have been told, blood pressure drugs are far from adverse-effect free. Ankle swelling, impotence, nightmares, cold extremities, fatigue, angioneurotic oedema (something I increasingly see), dry cough, the list goes on. These are not uncommon. In fact they are very common. ACE-inhibitors have recently been linked with depression and acute kidney failure.

However, in a weird twist of reality, I quite often come across research suggesting that when people take antihypertensive drugs, their quality of life does not actually get worse, it improves. This snippet was from a paper discussing the HOT (Hypertension Optimal Treatment) study:

"Although more intensive antihypertensive therapy is associated with a slight increase in subjective symptoms, it is nonetheless still associated with improvements in patients' well-being..."[57]

I find this statement impossible to believe. The main reason for my disbelief is that high blood pressure, in the vast majority of cases, causes absolutely no symptoms at all. For this very reason, it is often referred to as the 'silent killer.' On the other hand, taking blood pressure medication causes many adverse effects which are neither slight, nor subjective.

Here is a short personal testimonial from someone responding to a blog I wrote:

"From personal experience only on the use of beta-blockers, post quadruple by-pass operation, I was exceedingly ill for 5 years during which time I thought that each day was about to be my last. Five long years during which time I slept most days and slept at night. I was in a constant slumber and lacked energy. I also had severe neurological problems..."

These symptoms disappeared when she stopped taking the medication. Yet, when we take antihypertensive drugs, we are reliably informed that our quality of life will improve? So how does that happen, exactly? Of course the investigators who write such papers could never be accused of bias. Could they?

Referring to the study above, I just hit the first name on the list of authors. Ingela Wiklund. When the HOT paper was written she was working for AstraZeneca as Global Director of Outcome Research. The HOT study was funded by AstraZeneca, and used felodipine, which is an AstraZeneca drug.

Perhaps you can see a potential conflict of interest emerging here. Could her view on the adverse effects of felodipine possibly be biased in any way... by the fact that this study was done on an AstraZeneca drug, was funded, by AstraZeneca, and the lead author worked for AstraZeneca? I shall let you be the judge of that.

Let us compare and contrast this with a fascinating study that was done many years ago by a completely independent group of researchers.

They looked at the impact on quality of life on patients taking antihypertensives, which is pretty standard.

But they also did something I have not seen before, or since. They asked doctors what they thought about the quality of life of their patients on treatment. Then they asked the patients the same questions. Then, and I find this fascinating, they asked the patient's close relatives.

IS QUALITY OF LIFE IMPROVED, DOES IT STAY THE SAME, OR DOES IT GET WORSE ON BLOOD-PRESSURE LOWERING DRUGS?								
IMPROVED			STAYS THE SAME			WORSE		
Doctors	Patients	Relatives	Doctors	Patients	Relatives	Doctors	Patients	Relatives
75	36	1	0	32	0	0	7	74

"The questionnaire completed by relatives rated 19 patients (25 per cent) to have suffered mild adverse changes, 33 patients (45 per cent) to have had moderate adverse changes and 22 patients (30 per cent) severe adverse changes. The deteriorations were attributed to undue pre-occupation with sickness, decline in energy, general activity and sexual activity, and irritability."[58]

- 25% had mild adverse changes

- 45% had moderate adverse changes

- 30% severe adverse changes

As an exercise in proving that we see exactly what we want to see, I have never come across a more powerful paper. Every single doctor thought that the quality of life of their patients improved on drugs. All but one of the relatives thought that the quality of life of the patient got worse. In some cases much worse.

As for the patients, most of them said quality of life was the same – or better. What does this prove? I think I shall quote Robbie Burns on this matter: *"O would some power the giftie gie us to see ourselves as others see us."*

Robbie, you should have just asked your wife. She saw you better than anyone else.

In fact, the issue of doctors failing to notice adverse effects is widespread. For example, I believe that statins cause severe adverse effects, and that these are very common. When I ask patients about adverse effects most of them confirm at least one, usually more. Yet, many colleagues confidently inform me that they have never seen an adverse effect from a statin they have prescribed. Ever.

I suspect it may be the way you ask the question.

This form of words *'How are you getting on with your statin... fine... jolly good?'* Will probably result in the answer... *'fine, doctor, no problems at all.'*

I normally start with a little information. *'Statins can cause a lot of different effects, some of which you may put down to your age. For example, impotence, memory loss, aches and pains in the muscles, irritation and anger, rashes and suchlike. Have you noticed any of these?'*

If the patient comes in with a partner, I can usually see a light-bulb going off inside their heads as sudden realisation dawns. Yes, it's the statin. Now, you could say that I was leading the witness. Perhaps I am. I would say that I am giving them permission to talk about concerns.

On the other hand, I have heard literally hundreds of stories from patients who make it clear to me that their doctor does not have the slightest interest in discussing such things. Very often they try to shut the discussion down. Sometimes in a very blunt manner.

'Well, it's better than dying of a heart attack.' Or some other such pleasantry.

Which, in its way, is also a form of leading the witness... into a darkened cell, never to talk of such dreadful things as adverse effects ever again. No wonder the vast majority of patients stop taking their statins after two years – without telling their doctor. A splendid state of affairs. They just keep collecting their repeat subscription.

Anyway. Where was I? Getting back to the linear model again. This model takes all data points at blood pressures from around 90 mmHg to 190 mmHg and by using a clever mathematical equation, smoothes everything out. This creates an aesthetically pleasing line that rises from bottom left to top right of the page.

If you believe that this model is correct, then it follows that the blood pressure can be lowered from almost any level, to any lower level, and benefit will occur. You don't need to do a study to prove it, just feed the figures in, and the answer comes out.

Just one slight teeny, weeny, problem. If you analyse the data used to create the model, you find that the whole thing is nonsense, in fact *'it MUST be false.'*

Blood-pressure lowering tablets have many different effects that make interpreting the results from the clinical trials almost impossible.

The final reason – at least the final reason that I am going to talk about in this book – as to why the linear model is wrong, is because it relies on the assumption that all blood pressure drugs have one effect on cardiovascular disease, and one effect only. Lowering the blood pressure. Nothing else that these drugs do has the slightest impact on cardiovascular health.

To quote from an article in the *BMJ*

"... all the classes of blood-pressure lowering drugs have a similar effect in reducing CHD events and stroke for a given reduction in blood pressure so excluding material pleiotropic effects."[59]

'Pleiotropic effects' sounds highly scientific. However, it just means, the additional effects of a drug that are different from its central function. This is something that almost all drugs do – to a greater or lesser extent. Aspirin, for example, started life as a painkiller, then an anti-inflammatory, then it was used to prevent heart attacks and strokes. Now it is being used to protect against cancer.

Thalidomide started life as an anti sickness tablet during pregnancy. You will probably be aware that it encountered major problems in this role, but it is being used nowadays as an anti-cancer drug. Desmopressin, which can be used for bedwetting in children, is also used to treat haemophilia. Two conditions that you would not necessarily think were related in any way. Of course, they aren't, but a single drug has benefits in both.

Viagra and drugs of unintended consequences

Now to move the discussion somewhat closer to blood-pressure lowering by looking at Viagra. This drug began life as a treatment for angina. It was being tested for potential toxicity in healthy human volunteers when an interesting side-effect emerged. Yes, it improved erections. Cue handbrake turn and rapid change of marketing plan. The rest, as they say, is history.

Viagra was then found to have significant effects in pulmonary hypertension, which is one of the things that can kill you, if you develop altitude sickness. So mountaineers use it. It also stops them falling off mountains at night... (joke). Nowadays, Viagra is also used to treat patients with pulmonary hypertension at sea level. It is marketed under the name Revatio for this condition.

It can also be used in Raynaud's disease, as it helps to open up the small arteries supplying blood to the fingers, or toes. To the untrained eye, these effects may all seem pretty much unconnected. In reality they are all tightly bound together by one, single mechanism. It is, as follows. Viagra increases the production of nitric oxide (NO) in blood vessels or the walls of blood vessels.

Louis Ignarro, together with two colleagues, managed to isolate NO, to prove that it was an endothelial relaxing factor, and won the Nobel Prize for doing so. NO also has another critical effect in cardiovascular disease. It is the most powerful anticoagulant known to man. Which makes sense, as you don't want blood clots forming on top the endothelial cells that line artery walls.

Viagra has a multitude of different effects all around the body. It also lowers the blood pressure pretty effectively. As effectively as almost any other antihypertensive agent.

If we were to prescribe Viagra as an antihypertensive, which is entirely possible, and it were found reduce the risk of heart disease and stroke, which effect do you think would be responsible for the benefit? The blood-pressure lowering, or the anticoagulant effect? Or something else?

Aspirin and Viagra are far from unique in having many, many, different effects around the body. The simple fact is that, when you look around at the drugs commonly used in BP lowering, they *all* do many, many, different things throughout the cardio vascular system. BP lowering is often only one of them.

Ace-inhibitors, for example, a widely used antihypertensive agent, also raise NO, as do statins, and statins also lower the blood pressure.

"We found that statins lower both systolic and diastolic blood pressure, and that the effect extends to patients with pre-hypertension, with normal blood pressure, and persons not on blood-pressure lowering medication."

According to a news release from study researcher Beatrice Golomb, MD, PhD.[60]

Well, if statins raise NO, they must also lower blood pressure. So, this wasn't really a very surprising finding. Let me think about this for a moment. Statins raise NO and lower blood pressure. Could their benefits on CVD (in the very small group of people for whom they have any benefit

– men of a certain age who've already had a heart attack) possibly be due to these effects, and not cholesterol lowering... no, surely not.

Time, now to return to the statement from the *BMJ*:

"... all the classes of blood-pressure lowering drugs have a similar effect in reducing CHD events and stroke for a given reduction in blood pressure so excluding material pleiotropic effects."

This just is not true. Not even remotely. To quote the researchers from a major BP lowering study done at the turn of the millennium, the ALLHAT study. *"Blood pressure reduction is an **inadequate** surrogate marker for health benefits in hypertension."*

This study also showed a dramatic difference between alpha blockers and diuretics with, essentially, no difference in blood pressure reduction.

So great was the difference that a significant part of this study had to be terminated because those on the alpha-blockers were dying at a far higher rate than those on diuretic. At exactly the same blood pressure. The ALLHAT: interim results; ACC meeting (late breaking clinical trial results Anaheim CA March 15, 2000).

Here from the Cochrane collaboration: *"We cannot assume that drugs which are equivalent in lowering blood pressure will prove to be equally effective in reducing morbidity and mortality."*[61]

Here from an editorial in the *Journal of the American Medical Association*: *"Drugs that lower the blood pressure by about the same amount have very different outcomes."*[62]

HOPE (Heart Outcomes Prevention Evaluation) study demonstrated that,

"ACE inhibitors provided diverse and profound cardiovascular benefits, with only trivial differences in blood pressure between the treatment and control groups."[63]

I could quote this stuff for hundreds of pages. The reality is that different blood-pressure lowering agents have significantly different effects on outcomes – and these effects are completely and utterly independent of their effects on lowering blood pressure. This phenomenon was, in fact, first seen in the MRC study, where beta-blockers and diuretics lowered the blood pressure by the same amount, and had significantly different outcomes.

So far I have only mentioned the potentially positive pleiotropic effects of antihypertensive agents, but the effects can be negative as well as positive. For example, beta-blockers can cause diabetes, and diabetes increases the risk of heart disease.

Even with this overwhelming evidence to the contrary we are still supposed to believe that the *only* effect that blood-pressure lowering drugs have is on lowering blood pressure. Frankly, this is the most utter nonsense.

So, you might think, how can anyone manage to state that: *"all the classes of blood-pressure lowering drugs have a similar effect in reducing CHD events and stroke for a given reduction in blood pressure."*

Well, you need to put quotes like this in context. The context here is that this quote comes from an article by Professors Law and Wald. These two created the concept of a Polypill, of which you may have heard.

The Polypill started life as the concept of a single pill containing a low dose statin, three blood-pressure lowering drugs, aspirin and folic acid. A combination which they have promoted ruthlessly for many years now.

They also patented it. Which means that, if the Polypill were to be widely used, they would become richer than Croesus. In short they have a gigantic sky-scraping financial conflict of interest lurking in the background. Quelle surprise.

The simple fact here is this. If you are going to stick three low dose antihypertensive agents into a pill, you also have to argue that this combination, by acting together, will lower the blood pressure effectively. Also, that it is *only* their blood-pressure lowering effects that matter. No complications with pleiotropic effects can be allowed.

Because if this were not true, then the Polypill concept could not work without further testing each antihypertensive for pleiotropic effects, and then a review of how these pleiotropic effects might work together, or cancel each other out. That would require hundreds of millions to be spent on new research.

(Law and Wald have already removed aspirin and folic acid from the tablet, as the latest research had found that neither agent provides significant benefits in CVD. Despite this, all their other calculations about the benefits of the Polypill remain solid and inarguable. Ho, ho).

But how, you may ask, did they manage to prove this statement? *"All the classes of blood-pressure lowering drugs have a similar effect in reducing CHD events and stroke for a given reduction in blood pressure."*

And get it published?

Well, they played the assumptions game. In this game, before you do a statistical analysis you define how you are going to do it, and make various assumptions about the data. In this case they started here:

"Participants: 464,000 people defined into three mutually exclusive categories: participants with no history of vascular disease, a history of CHD, or a history of stroke."

Now, you can read that, and shrug your shoulders. So what? You may cry. But pay close attention. Law and Wald have decreed that people with no history of vascular disease, a history of CHD, or a history of stroke, are three mutually exclusive categories. Oh, really. In what way, exactly, are these groups mutually exclusive?

Just think about this for a moment. What they are saying is that, if you have a history of CHD, you CANNOT have a history of stroke, as these are mutually exclusive categories. Ask any doctor on the planet earth and they will tell you that stroke and heart disease are so closely related as to be, in many cases, indistinguishable from each other. They are different sides of the same coin. Which is not exactly surprising as the underlying pathology is, in the majority of cases, precisely the same.

It is why they are both filed under the general header cardiovascular disease (CVD). Not only is the underlying pathology exactly the same, the factors causing both are also almost exactly the same. If you do primary or secondary prevention studies in cardiovascular medicine, it is to attempt to prevent both strokes and heart disease.

Furthermore, it is completely ridiculous to claim that those with no history of vascular disease constitute another exclusive group. If you are a seventy year old heavy smoker with type 2 diabetes and high blood pressure, you are at a very high risk of having both a heart attack and stroke – even if you have not had one yet. You could well have extensive atherosclerosis in every major artery in your body, but if you haven't been diagnosed with it then you will have 'no history'.

In short, if you start your analysis by making wildly inaccurate assumptions, such as claiming that people with a history of CHD, stroke and no history of vascular diseases are mutually exclusive populations, then you are starting from a place that has no known basis in any medical reality. Or any other form of reality.

At which point, any conclusions you draw, however clever your statistical tests, are nonsense. You may be glad to know that I am not going to dissect this paper in any further depth. I just want you to be aware that, like the best conjuring tricks, in many medical papers the trick happened a long time before you think the magician has started doing anything.

'Pick an assumption, any assumption. No... not that one... this one.'

'Oh the one where people with strokes and heart attacks are mutually exclusive populations.'

Yes, that one... '

'...Bong!'

Yet, despite this, and all the other reasons that I have mentioned, the belief in this model remains unquestioned. The magnificent clothes of the Emperor, stitched together with such care, with so many reputations dependent on everyone gasping in awe. So much money spent, so much money to be spent in the future from creating even more resplendent garments.

If the linear model were to be declared wrong, the entire edifice of blood-pressure lowering would collapse, which would represent a major catastrophe for all sorts of people. Mainly, perhaps, the pharmaceutical industry.

Key points about the linear model and surrogate end-points:

1. The linear model was created from the Framingham data, but when you analyse it, the model does not fit the data. So the entire basis on which blood pressure is lowered was wrong, and remains wrong.

2. Because there are no placebo-controlled studies done any more, it is impossible to know if lowering blood pressure with different drugs, or combinations of drugs, is any better than placebo – and may be worse. We rely on the model – see point 1.

3. Different blood-pressure lowering drugs must have, and do have, different effects on heart attacks and strokes, yet the model states that they do not.

If I were to summarize the entire area of blood-pressure lowering, and the research done here, I would refer back to the Professor Ionnadis view of research.

"Moreover, for many current scientific fields, claimed research findings may often be simply accurate measures of the prevailing bias."

J Ionnadis

The prevailing bias here is that the linear model is true, and we can use surrogate end-points to calculate benefit. Consciously, or unconsciously, or financially, all research is adapted to fit into this prevailing paradigm. Pity that it happens to be wrong.

CHAPTER SIX

Challenges to the status quo
are crushed – and how!

"Why do people insist on defending their ideas and opinions with such fe-rocity, as if defending honour itself? What could be easier to change than an idea?"

J.G. Farrell. *The Siege of Krishnapur*

I think it was Jeremy Paxman, of BBC fame, who was supposed to say to himself, before every interview with a politician: 'Why is this lying bastard lying to me now?'

Nowadays, I am afraid to say, I approach medical research papers in much the same way as Jeremy Paxman approaches an interview. I rarely look at a headline and think, jolly good, here is an honest attempt to get at the truth. I think... OK, what's going on here? Why have these people written this? What's their agenda?

More recently I have started to scan the title of a scientific paper, read what it says, and wonder if it even reflects the findings of the study. You may believe that this, surely, cannot be questioned. Surely, the title of a scientific paper must be a short, yet accurate, summary of what was actually found. Ah... no.

Here, for example is the title of a paper looking at dairy food con-sumption and heart disease. "Is dairy product consumption associated with the incidence of CHD?"[64]

Now, reading that, what is your immediate thought? You think they are asking a rhetorical question, and that this study probably demon-strates that eating a lot of dairy products does increase the risk of heart disease. Well, the results were that:

117

*"Women with higher intake of **low-fat** cheese and **non-fat** milk seem to have a higher risk of incident CHD. This needs further investigation considering recent evidence of cardiovascular benefits from certain dairy fat."*

So, why didn't they call their study. 'Low-fat *dairy product consumption increases the risk of CHD.'* Also, please note the word 'seem' here. This word pops up all the time when people find things they don't much like the look of.

Is being overweight bad for you?

For many years I have been studying excess weight and obesity. One of the key questions I set out to answer for myself was the following. How dangerous is it to overall health? I am fully aware that we are bombarded with the message that being overweight and obese causes massive health problems such as, diabetes, and heart disease, and cancer and... well, you get the picture.

I don't think there is much doubt that exceedingly obese individuals suffer from significant health problems, which will wipe several years off their life expectancy. But I wanted to know the answer to a question that I once thought might be quite simple to answer. At what point does being 'overweight' create significant health problems?

I started off by looking at the body mass index (BMI) classification. As you may know, the BMI is a calculation based on your weight, in kilograms, divided by your height squared, in metres. BMI = kg/m^2. This took over from the ponderosity index about fifty years ago.

Although the classifications do vary a little, these are the generally accepted boundaries:

Underweight	BMI < 18.5
Normal weight	BMI 18.5-24.9
Overweight	BMI 25-29.9
Obese	BMI > 30

You would think that, having categorised weight into four basic types, it would be natural to assume that being of 'normal weight' is good for your health. Whereas being underweight is bad for your health, as is being overweight and obese. Otherwise, why on Earth would these categories exist?

Ignoring the underweight category for the moment, the clear assumption behind having an 'overweight' classification is that a BMI above 25 marks the point at which your weight starts to cause damage. Within this context, it should come as no surprise to find a major study in the *Journal of the American Medical Association* with the title: "Excess deaths associated with underweight, overweight, and obesity."[65]

This title would appear to confirm everything that everybody already knows about weight and health. However, if you choose to actually read the paper itself, here is a curious statement from the results section. *"Overweight was **not** associated with excess mortality."*

(I put the word *not* in bold).

Strange... try to fit those words into the title of the paper. I suspect you can't.

In fact, although this statement was somewhat less misleading than the title of the paper, it is still not an accurate reflection of their findings. What they actually found was that being overweight was associated with a significantly *reduced* mortality. Otherwise known as increased life expectancy. I will put it another way, because you may not have quite understood what you just read.

Those who were overweight lived the longest.

I shall repeat this, so that there can be no possible misunderstanding

Those who were overweight lived the longest.

Why, then, does the title explicitly state that excess deaths are associated with being overweight? The data from this study are unequivocal. Those who were overweight lived longer than people in any other weight category. And although association cannot prove causation, a lack of association does disprove causation.

The researchers themselves cannot possibly have failed to understand what they found. It also seems extraordinarily unlikely that they somehow slipped up in writing the title... and the abstract... and the conclusions.

You do not send a paper to the *Journal of the American Medical Association* (*JAMA*), one of the most prestigious medical journals in the world, without reviewing it many, many, times. Then thinking long and hard about what you are going to call it. And after thinking long and hard about it, they gave it a title which clearly states that being overweight is associated with an excess death rate.

Interesting.

Why would anyone do this? At this point I am only speculating, but bear with me whilst I do so. Within the world of obesity research the current view is that being overweight is bad for your health. Most doctors absolutely believe this to be true. In fact, almost everyone in the world knows this to be true.

Even the mighty Wikipedia confirms it:

"The generally accepted view is that being overweight causes similar health problems to obesity, but to a lesser degree. Adams et al. estimated that the risk of death increases by 20 to 40 percent among overweight people, and the Framingham heart study found that being overweight at age 40 reduced life expectancy by three years."[66]

(It seems churlish to point out to Wikipedia that the risk of death always remains stubbornly at one. You cannot increase, or decrease it unless you are James Bond).

Moving on. The authoritative patient website *patient.co.uk* makes the following statement on obesity and overweight.

"If you are obese or overweight, this means that you are carrying excess body fat. Being overweight or obese is not just about how you look. Over time, it means that you have an increased risk of developing various health problems."

In general you will find that the terms overweight and obesity are wrapped together as a kind of generally bad thing. Overweight is seen as a form of 'obesity lite.' Not quite as bad as being obese, but still bad.

The reality, however, is completely different. The majority of studies (Framingham aside) find that those with a BMI in the overweight category have the longest life span. The older you get, the more beneficial it is to be overweight. A major German meta-analysis in 2009 grudgingly came to this conclusion.

"The prevailing notion that overweight increases morbidity and mortality, as compared to so-called normal weight, is in need of further specification."[67]

Ah, yes, you cannot say that the prevailing notion is wrong. It is *"in need of further specification."* Whatever, exactly, that is supposed to mean. For those who like a graph, and I usually do, although I have avoided them up to now. Here is a major study from Canada.[68]

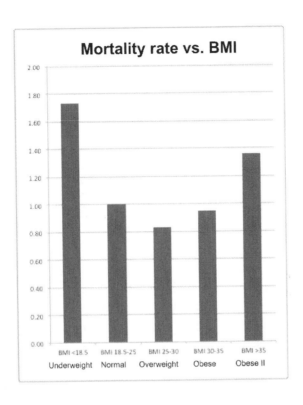

Mortality rate vs. BMI

In the words of the Authors

"Our results are similar to those from other recent studies, confirming that underweight and obesity class II+ are clear risk factors for mortality, and showing that when compared to the acceptable BMI category, overweight appears to be protective against mortality."

I love the word 'appears.' It is very similar to the word 'seemed'. They just cannot bring themselves to say that, overweight *is* protective against mortality. You may note that, in this study, even those in the obese category (BMI 30-35) had a lower mortality than those of 'normal' weight. That, however, is a discussion for another place. The main point I wanted to make here is the following.

The overwhelming belief in the medical community is that being overweight is bad for you. It causes a host of diseases, which will inevitably result in premature death. To state that being overweight means that you live longer, is the scientific equivalent of standing up and shouting that the Emperor is not actually wearing any clothes at all.

Thou shall not question

In the medical research world, those in positions of power do not take kindly to anyone daring to question the established order. Instead, they close ranks, and retaliate.

"When I entered medicine, I did not realize that there was such intense pressure to conform. But we learn early on that there is a decorum to medicine, a politeness. A hidden curriculum teaches us not to disturb the status quo. We are trained to defer to authority, not to question it. We depend on powerful individuals and organizations and are taught that success does not often come to those who ask uncomfortable questions or suggest new ways of providing care.

"The sense of danger that we feel when we question authority is not unfounded. Those who ask difficult questions or challenge conventional wisdom are often isolated. They may find few opportunities to speak and their writings may not be welcome. Compliance with normative behaviour may be forced by fear of recrimination. In some cases, junior faculty may fear that support from mentors will be withdrawn or promotions denied.

"I have seen evidence of many such efforts to coerce conformity of opinion and behaviour. I have heard of junior faculty who were told that questioning key assumptions of the field, even with evidence, would result in threats to funding and support.

"A Note to my younger colleagues – be brave."

Harlan M. Krumholz, MD, SM (Editorial in *Circulation*)

"Unfortunately, in the academic world—where much of today's scientific innovation takes place—researchers are encouraged to maintain the status quo and not 'rock the boat.' This mentality is pervasive, affecting all aspects of scientific research from idea generation to funding to the training of the next generation of scientists."

Fred Southwick[69]

What happens if your research threatens to upset the status quo? What would you do? Go with it, and damn the consequences? Or fudge it?

Perhaps I can help you to make up your mind by providing a few examples of what happens to those who challenge dogma, and damn the consequences. Starting with Peter Gøtzsche.

He is a respected researcher, professor, and director of the Nordic Cochrane collaboration. He has been studying the benefits and harms of breast cancer screening for over 15 years, alongside other activities. He has no axe to grind – that I can see. He is very measured and meticulous in his research.

He has come to the view that the benefits of screening have been greatly hyped, and that potential downsides have been deliberately downplayed. He is highly critical of the way in which information on breast screening has been presented to women, with no possible downsides.

For saying such things he has been relentlessly attacked by the pro-screening lobby. The primary weapon used is the 'you're killing my patients' ploy. Here is one such example of an attack. It is a letter that was written about Gøtzsche. He was sent it by a friend and colleague who was included in the circulation list, and Gøtzsche included it in his book *Mammography Screening*:

"What is remarkable to me is that this man G [Peter Gøtzsche] calls himself a scientist since he obviously and knowingly ignores the scientific method in order to further his own agenda, whatever that may be. I cannot believe he is so intellectually deficient that he cannot grasp the plethora of evidence that so strongly supports the benefit of screening. What then drives him so blindly in his crusade to convince us all that the world is flat?

*"To become infamous as a contrarian, standing lonely on the curvature of the earth as he denies it is spinning under his feet? Or is it something even more petty? An all-consuming hatred and jealousy of Laslo Tabar, whose impeccable trial facilitated by meticulous record keeping and a socialist society provides a setting unparalleled in the world for a scientific trial? What is tragic and makes G's ravings sinister is that **I am sure his influence has resulted in women's unnecessary deaths... Etc."** (My emphasis).*

Accusing people of killing women is pretty down and dirty. But as Professor Michael Baum, mentioned earlier, has made clear. *"Any who dares challenge the sacred cow of screening has a terrible time."* He is right.

Moving on to an even more contentious area, HIV and AIDS. For some time I have been interested in the work of Peter Duesberg. Someone you have almost certainly never heard of. Here is a little snippet from his biography.

"Peter H. Duesberg, Ph.D. is a professor of Molecular and Cell Biology at the University of California, Berkeley. He isolated the first cancer gene through his work on retroviruses in 1970, and mapped the genetic structure of these viruses. This, and his subsequent work in the same field, resulted in his election to the National Academy of Sciences in 1986. He is also the recipient of a seven-year Outstanding Investigator Grant from the National Institutes of Health..."[70]

This much is true, and uncontested. On the surface he is a highly respected researcher. At least he was, once. Duesberg is now famous, or infamous, for his hypothesis that HIV is not the cause of AIDS. He makes an interesting case, and there are many other scientists who agree with him. Including the man who developed the Polymerase Chain Reaction (PCR) test, and won the Nobel Prize for doing so, Kary Mullis. PCR is *the* test used to find the HIV virus.

I don't know if Duesberg is right or wrong, and it is an argument that I am not entering, as it is a very complex and specialised area (and I know I will be attacked for even daring to mention his name). But that is not the point I am making here. The point I am making is that he, an eminent expert in his field, has gone against the mainstream view of the 'experts' in this field. This has resulted in him being savagely attacked. And when I say savagely, I mean savagely.

An on-line article by Jeanne Bergman for AIDStruth.org is the best concentrated example of character assassination that I have ever come across. In this passage she has adapted a *Newsweek* article entitled "Newsweek exposes Duesberg's psychopathology", which was written by Interlandi:

"Interlandi describes how Duesberg has 'toiled in scientific purgatory' at Berkeley. An embarrassment to the University, he has been relegated to a crummy little lab in a shabby building, with no grant funding, no promising graduate students, and no respect from anyone—including other cancer researchers working on aneuploidy. He is no longer allowed to teach.

"Duesberg clearly understands that this follows from his failed theory that HIV is harmless. Interlandi identifies in him a core conflict between two equally disturbing character traits: 'he craves a return to respectability, [and] he refuses to cede any ground to his adversaries.' (See AIDS truth's article about his malignant narcissism.)

"But Duesberg seems unable to grasp that the contempt is the result of his refusal to accept the conclusive scientific evidence that HIV is the cause of AIDS, and of his persistent proselytizing of his disproven claims about HIV, AIDS and antiretrovirals, which has caused hundreds of thousands of unnecessary deaths, particularly in South Africa.

"The Newsweek profile touches on the formative impact of Nazism on Duesberg, who grew up a privileged Catholic in fascist Germany, and the resulting attitudes he holds toward people who aren't heterosexual white men. He degrades women and developmentally disabled people (both lack 'all the IQ genes,' he told Interlandi, 'half joking').

"He calls black people 'Schwartzes' (the German N-word) and gays 'homos,' and describes both as evolutionary failures. His assistant calls these 'gaffes,' and says of Duesberg: 'He's just from a different era, when people actually talked like that.' Actually, only Nazis and other racists, homophobes and eugenicists talked like that. Decent people of any age didn't, and don't."[71]

Now, you can disagree with Duesberg if you like, and many people do. You can marshal your scientific arguments and engage him in debate. Or, you can do what is usually done to those who hold ideas that do not fit with that of the authorities. You attack. In this case you call him a homophobic, racist, narcissistic, nazi-sympathising, mass-murderer – one who also casually insults the disabled.

That, I think, is the royal flush of insults. What's missing? I think the author passed over the opportunity to call Duesberg a paedophile. But it was only a short article; you can only get so many insults into three hundred words.

Exactly the same depressing and horrible game is played in other 'sensitive' areas. Here is a personal testimony from a Dutch medical journalist Melchior Meijer about the way he has been treated. The passage that follows is from a Dutch on-line discussion forum:

"My name is Melchior Meijer. I'm a medical reporter for several magazines and newspapers in The Netherlands. Reporting about the many obvious flaws in the cholesterol hypothesis, shedding light on the biologically plausible adverse consequences of statin therapy, is as close to 21st century blasphemy as a medical journalist can come.

"I experienced this in 2004, when I wrote an article about statins in a national newspaper. In the article, several doctors and scientists expressed well founded doubts about the safety of statin therapy in the general population. I also presented a few 'anecdotal' cases of statin induced harm, which were extremely easy to find.

"The medical establishment reacted in fury and started an aggressive media offensive. Carefully avoiding the arguments in my article, they used their authority to hang me out on TV as a liar, a potential mass murderer. They called for 'official measures' to prevent naive journalists from making similar 'tragic mistakes' in the future.

"They also took me to the Press Court, but they didn't reckon with the fact that the Press Court checks facts and figures. The Court did an investigation and decided that I had just done my job, observing and questioning. [As an aside: the chief of my newspaper, born into a family of influential physicians, was not happy with the Court's decision. He had already apologized on television for 'this tragic mistake'.]

"After this, statin users started calling and mailing to the media, always reporting the same symptoms: various degrees of (muscle pain) and loss of muscle mass, exhaustion, personality changes and amnesia. But my colleagues didn't like to take up this serious issue. That is, until last March when the TV-colleagues of TROS Radar, a consumer programme with an average of 2 million watchers (we have 16 million inhabitants), took up the subject.

"Dutch cardiologist Dr Paul de Groot expressed his doubts about cholesterol as a causal factor, and postulated that statins sometimes do more harm than good, especially in primary prevention. Dr Uffe Ravnskov, who by the way was honoured yesterday with the prestigious Leo Prize for independent science, pointed out the many flaws in the cholesterol hypothesis.

"The programme also interviewed people who had experienced devastating side effects from statins, which quickly disappeared upon discontinuation – although sometimes they did not. I was on the programme to explain how Unilever had succeeded in keeping an unfavourable article about its cholesterol lowering spread Flora out of the press.

"When the shit hits the fan...

"My time is limited, so I will make it short. Radar was vigorously attacked from all directions. Professors Martijn Katan and John Kastelein used various media outlets to shamelessly fire irrelevant, slanderous attacks on Dr Ravnskov. As usual, they did not address any of the scientific arguments. Radar invited Katan and Kastelein for a public debate with Drs. Ravsnkov and Kendrick, but they declined.

"The Dutch Cardiologists Association, together with the Healthcare Inspectorate – and this is critical – announced official guidelines for medical journalists who plan to cover 'delicate medical matters.'"

To be fair, Melchior has only been accused of being a 'mass murderer and a liar.' Not a homophobe, racist, nazi-sympathising, misogynist. He got off rather lightly.

More recently I helped an Australian journalist, Dr Maryanne Demasi, working for the Australian Broadcasting Corporation, to put together two programmes: one questioning the diet-heart-cholesterol hypothesis; the other challenging the over prescribing of statins.

The attempt at censorship started even before the programmes aired. Professor Emily Banks, chair of the Advisory Committee on the Safety of Medicines wrote to ABC 'in a private capacity' (not sure how that works) and claimed "If people stop using their statins or if they don't start them when they should be, it's very likely that it will result in death."

The programme aired and then the messy stuff hit the fan. The pharma lobby went into overdrive. Numerous claims were lodged with the Australian broadcasting standards body. Several months later their investigation concluded that there had been one breach of one code on one occasion. 16 other complaints were not upheld. Corrective action was recommended for this one breach. So what did ABC do? They pulled both programmes. The reporter was subject to defamation, accused of "killing people" and one Sydney cardiologist declared "ABC has blood on its hands."

There was much more in this vein – as totally expected. In fact, I blogged about this, and 'made the following prediction[72]. Here is what I wrote:

"History, you see, does repeat itself, and so I can predict what now happens in Australia. There will be calls to bring in 'official guideline for medical journalists who plan to cover delicate medical matters.' This is also known as press censorship. It has been popular in various dictatorships over the years. Currently, North Korea is the best place to see this in action."

Lo and behold...

The Parliament of New South Wales Committee on the Health Care Complaints Commission launched an "Inquiry into the promotion of false or misleading health-related information or practices." The terms of reference were as follows:

"That the Committee on the Health Care Complaints Commission inquire into and report on possible measures to address the promotion of unscientific health related information or practices which may be detrimental to individual or public health. The Inquiry will focus on individuals who are not recognised health practitioners, and organisations that are not recognised health service providers.

"The Committee will have particular regard to:

a. *The publication and/or dissemination of false or misleading health related information that may cause general community mistrust of, or anxiety toward, accepted medical practice;*

b. *The publication and/or dissemination of information that encourages individuals or the public to unsafely refuse preventative health measures medical treatments, or cures;*

c. *The promotion of health related activities and/or provision of treatment that departs from accepted medical practice which may be harmful to individual or public health;*

d. *The adequacy of the powers of the Health Care Complaints Commission to investigate such organisations or individuals;*

e. *The capacity appropriateness and effectiveness of the Health Care Complaints Commission to take enforcement action against such organisations or individuals; and*

f. *any other related matter."*

What is particularly sinister is point b)

"The publication and/or dissemination of information that encourages individuals or the public to unsafely refuse preventative health measures medical treatments, or cures."

Well, well, well. God bless free speech and personal choice. Do you think the Australian Government will confiscate and burn this book, and put anyone in jail who reads it? This new law is most certainly going to frighten any journalist away from covering the views of all scientific sceptics, forever.

Well, before it is banned in Australia, I will include a few passages from an article in the *BMJ*, 2nd November 2013. It was called: "Overdiagnosis: when good intentions meet vested interests."[73] Written by Iona Heath, a past president of the Royal College of General Practitioners in the UK.

"Underpinned by webs of financial imperatives and conflicted interests, overdiagnosis and overtreatment have become disturbingly pervasive within contemporary medicine and are now deeply embedded within healthcare systems around the world. They have permeated and polluted the drug and medical technology industry, medical research and regulatory bodies, clinical practice, payment systems, guideline production, and national healthcare systems..."

She goes on to say.

"Overdiagnosis and overtreatment have at least four serious ethical implications. The first is the extent of harm to the individuals caused by being labelled as being at risk or as having a disease based entirely on numbers or other aberrant investigations and the unnecessary fear that this can engender which in itself can undermine health and wellbeing.

"The second involves the direct relation between overtreatment and undertreatment, because whenever a diagnosis is broadened, attention and resources are inevitably redirected and shifted away from those most severely affected. The third

concerns the potential of overdiagnosis and overtreatment to render a healthcare system based on social solidarity unviable because of the escalating costs involved.

"The fourth is the way in which biotechnical activity marginalises and obscures the socioeconomic causes of ill health. So what of politics? Back in 1964, the German American political theorist, Herbert Marcuse wrote: 'Totalitarian is not only a terroristic political coordination of society, but also a non-terroristic economic technical coordination which operates through the manipulation of needs by vested interest.' This is what large tracts of our healthcare systems have become: a non-terroristic economic technical coordination that operates through the manipulation of needs by vested interests."

Goodness me, I think Iona Heath's article definitely comes under parts a) b) and c) of that Australian document. She is most certainly saying we are over-diagnosing and over-treating. This means that she is encouraging individuals and the wider public to mistrust accepted medical practice. Perhaps the New South Wales Govt. should arrest Dr Iona Heath, and sue the *BMJ* for publishing reactionary and dangerous articles.

Oh, they don't actually mean this.

No, what they mean is that they are going to pick on relatively powerless individuals, and journalists, and stomp them into silence. As they did with Melchior Meijer in the Netherlands. This, of course, is where State Censorship usually begins... and where does it end? Well, we know where it ends:

First they came for the communists,
and I didn't speak out because I wasn't a communist.

Then they came for the socialists,
and I didn't speak out because I wasn't a socialist.

Then they came for the trade unionists,
and I didn't speak out because I wasn't a trade unionist.

Then they came for me,
and there was no one left to speak for me

Do you think this is a massive over-reaction? Do I really believe that we are heading for some form of totalitarian state, where dissent against the medical 'experts' will be punishable by imprisonment? Well, yes, I do. We are already in a situation where doctors who fail to follow the dreaded 'guidelines' can be sued, or dragged in front of the General Medical Council, and struck off. Thus losing their job, and income.

I thought I would include another example, one of many libellous attacks that Dr Uffe Ravnskov had endured for proposing that raised cholesterol levels are not the cause of coronary heart disease.

"Dear Mister Ravnskov,

"I read with interest your letter in the BMJ, in the 20 September issue of 2008.

"You state that cholesterol has nothing to do with the incidence of cardio-vascular disease in individuals with familial hypercholesterolemia. You also state that the effect of statin therapy is grossly overstated and that women do not benefit and that the benefits are easily outweighed by side effects.

"If this was [sic] a joke, I could have laughed about your statements heartily, but they are in fact criminal and bordering on the insane. I am aware of the fact that you have advised a mother with a daughter suffering from FH to feed her organic vegetables and that the link between cholesterol and early heart disease did not exist in FH but was in fact due to a tendency to blood-clotting.

"I suggest you read the work that my colleague Dr Sijbrands and myself [sic] published in the BMJ in 2001[xi] as well as the article published in BMJ last week. I also suggest you take good notice of the JUPITER results that I published together with Dr Paul Ridker in the NEJM last week. These 3 studies completely contradict all of your ridiculous contentions. In fact, I insist that you refrain from any advice to any patient anymore. You are lucky not to live in the Netherlands. I would have dragged you to court. I have cared for patients with familial hyper-cholesterolemia since 1987 and I have seen the terrible devastation that this disease can bring to families. I have also seen what the introduction of statins has done and your nonsense is creating an anger in me that I have not experienced for a long time."

Professor Dr J.J.P. Kastelein

Joyce Jansen

P.A. to John J.P. Kastelein, MD, PhD

Professor of Medicine

I keep a file of such attacks – including the ones that I regularly receive. Here is just one recent one, following a blog article that I wrote:

---

xi I find it amusing that Kastelein quotes this study, as it clearly demonstrated that people with Familial Hypercholesterolaemia (FH) live slightly longer than those without FH – maybe he thought no-one would notice.

"Dr Kendrick

"There is undoubtedly deceit, subterfuge, corruption and laziness in the world of medical research.

"I am a specialist anaesthetist with a sub speciality interest in vascular anaesthesia at a large tertiary medical centre. I am a clinical anaesthetist with no research activities, not beholden to any pharmaceutical company nor ever in receipt of gifts from such companies.

"I am very familiar with all the studies in question and was appalled, like the majority of practitioners, at the events surrounding Dr Poldermans research and the extent of his deceit and malpractice.

"However your 'blog' is irresponsible, dangerous and scaremongering. It will cause many who read it unnecessary anxiety and stress. It is devoid of fact and evidence and will do nothing to further the debate.

"There is so much worthy of discussion regarding the whole affair and so many lessons to be learnt. You do not attempt to do that, rather you choose reckless hyperbole and sensationalist superficial headlines.

"It is absurd to suggest that you can say with any certainty the potential harm done by his fraudulent research. To casually go on record as saying that you can almost certainly say that 800,000 people have died is ridiculous. In doing so you confirm your real agenda, which is self-promotion and notoriety.

"People need doctors and they have a right to expect highly skilled ones. When doctors fail to behave professionally, apologies, debate, education and improvement are what is required. Polarising debate with nonsense hinders progress and intelligent discussion."

Blah, blah. Thanks very much for that.

I would like to say that such attacks don't bother me in the least. But when you can be accused of killing thousands of people by advising them not to take statins, it can be a little tricky merely to shrug your shoulders. Especially when you can be referred to the General Medical Council at any time, and struck off the medical register for 'bringing the medical profession into disrepute', as I mentioned before.

So, I would say to Harlan M. Krumholz that being brave is all very well, and noble. But being brave doesn't pay the mortgage. Also, if you want to climb the slippery pole in medical research, the best thing you can do is to stick very closely to the mainstream view. Or else you will very rapidly find yourself without funding. This is just the way this world works.

It is probably the way that the rest of the scientific world works as well, and always has been, but I can't be certain as I am primarily interested in medical research. However, a quote from Max Plank (the man who published Albert Einstein's special theory of relativity, against vociferous opposition by his editorial board), makes me feel that challenging the status quo has never been a great idea.

"Truth never triumphs – its opponents just die out. Science advances one funeral at a time."

Max Plank

So, to return to the question I posed quite a while ago now. Why did the authors choose this title for their paper?

"Excess deaths associated with underweight, overweight, and obesity."

I would suggest it is because, if they dared to write a paper with this title...

"Excess deaths associated with underweight, normal weight, and obesity."

...one of two things would have happened. Either the peer reviewers would have rejected it. Or, had it been published, their names would be mud in the world of obesity research.

My own belief is that the investigators thought to themselves – something along the lines of – we cannot possibly use such a title, it will cause an uproar. We would have to start advising people who are of 'normal' weight to gain weight if they want to live longer. This is going to sound incredibly... incredibly stupid. Our peers are going to go nuts. The public will say we have no idea what we are talking about. We keep changing our minds. Indeed.

So, I believe that they fudged. They gave the paper a title that would be acceptable to the obesity experts. They played down their own findings, and in the conclusions section, they didn't even mention the overweight category at all. Here, in their own words:

"Underweight and obesity, particularly higher levels of obesity, were associated with increased mortality relative to the normal weight category."

I may be wrong, they may not have been attacked – merely ignored. Not all attacks are overt and vicious; they do not need to be. Most of the pressure in the world of scientific research is exerted like some elaborate courtship dance whose rules can be opaque to the outside world. *'But we learn early on that there is a decorum to medicine, a politeness. A*

132

hidden curriculum teaches us not to disturb the status quo.' You only know you lost when you find yourself sitting outside in the cold rain, looking in through the windows at the happy dancing couples, and wondering what the hell just happened. But shame on you *JAMA* for not having the courage to propose a more appropriate title... what are you afraid of?

The part played by peer review

One of the best games played to ensure that the status quo is disturbed as little as possible, is the use of peer review. In this system you ask acknowledged 'experts' in areas of medicine to review papers that are sent in to your journals. Their job is then to decide if said papers are fit to publish. Of course, by definition, anyone who is an 'expert' in an area of medicine will be a supporter of whatever dogma holds sway. Most likely, their entire career was built on developing and supporting it.

Then, along comes a researcher in all their merry innocence, demonstrating that everything the current batch of experts believes is wrong. They happily send in their research paper to the *Journal of Very Important Research*. The Journal sends it off to their favourite experts... guess what the outcome is likely to be.

"Science is normally presented to the public as an enterprise based on scepticism and openness to new idea, in which evidence and argumentation are examined on their own merits. Trusting newcomers who present views that conflict with standard ideas may thus expect that their work will be given a prompt, fair, and inclusive analysis, being accepted if it passes scrutiny and being given detailed reasons why not.

"When, instead, their work is ignored, ridiculed, or rejected without explanation, they assume that there has been some sort of mistake, and often begin a search to find the 'right person': someone who fits the stereotype of the open-minded scientist. This can be a long search."

Brian Martin. *Strategies for Dissenting Scientists*

Even the editors of main journals themselves recognise that peer review may not be the best system ever devised by mankind. Here is what Richard Horton, the editor of *The Lancet*, has to say on the matter:

"The mistake, of course, is to have thought that peer review was any more than a crude means of discovering the acceptability — not the validity — of a new finding. Editors and scientists alike insist on the pivotal importance of peer review. We portray peer review to the public as a quasi-sacred process that helps

to make science our most objective truth teller. But we know that the system of peer review is biased, unjust, unaccountable, incomplete, easily fixed, often insulting, usually ignorant, occasionally foolish, and frequently wrong."

Ah yes, what a system: *"biased, unjust, unaccountable, incomplete, easily fixed, often insulting, usually ignorant, occasionally foolish, and frequently wrong."*[74]

Although it must be said that, if your aim is to stifle innovation and obliterate challenges to the status quo, peer review is *the* perfect system. Ask those with by far the most to lose if the current dogma is successfully overturned to make an objective decision as to the worth of controversial new research. Bong!

One of the only journals that did not have peer review was *Medical Hypotheses*. A journal at one time edited by Bruce Charlton (quoted earlier with reference to Zombie medicine). This journal was designed to promote novel hypothesis, and new ideas, and to challenge current thinking. (I had an article published in it a few years ago).

But Bruce Charlton made one of the two unforgivable current sins in medicine. He published an article by Duesberg, the evil 'aids denier.' A huge storm of protest ensued, with demands for retraction and heads to roll. The Spanish Inquisition rides again. Bruce Charlton refused, and stood his ground. The publishers told him to retract, or else. So he resigned in protest.

As a result of all this, the journal *Medical Hypotheses* is now peer reviewed, which must be the greatest oxymoron ever. Put forward a completely new idea and have it reviewed by your peers... And which peers would they be? The peers who had exactly the same, completely never thought of before idea, several years before. Ho, ho, you earthlings are so funny.

The end result of this sorry saga is that the only journal (catalogued and listed on Medline) that was willing to put forward new ideas was crushed for putting forward a new idea. In addition, an editor who was willing to take on mainstream thinking resigned – forced from the battlefield. Inflexible dogmatic thought 1: Innovation 0.

At this point I hope I have made it clear that it is *enormously* difficult to challenge the status quo – otherwise known as the view of the 'experts'. A few have managed over the years. Probably the most famous recent example would be Barry Marshall and Robin Warren who demonstrated that gastric ulcers were (mainly) caused by the bacterium helicobacter pylori. This flew in the face of the presiding paradigm that gastric ulcers were due to stress, which caused increased stomach acid production.

When Barry Marshall demonstrated the presence of bacteria on pathology slides to 'experts' they claimed the bacteria weren't actually there. They were just an artefact. Yes, when people really don't want to see a thing, they will actually refuse to believe the evidence of their own eyes. This reminds me of a little tale about a chap called Galileo.

Would you, or I, have carried on at this point? I would like to think I would, but when the entire establishment is intent on ridiculing you...

"For years, Barry Marshall and Robin Warren faced ridicule and hostility from the academic and industrial scientific communities for claiming that ulcers could be caused by a bacterial infection. After years of dogged pursuit, even to the point of swallowing a culture of Helicobacter pylori to show that it could infect the stomach lining, the researchers proved their case, changed medical thinking radically, and were awarded the Nobel Prize for Medicine or Physiology this year for their endeavours."[75]

A question that often disturbs me is the following. How many Marshall and Warrens are there who were right, but gave up in the face of massive hostility and ridicule? I suppose we can never know. Or, even worse, how many Marshall and Warrens took one look at the battlefield and decided not even to bother entering in the first place?

I find this one of the biggest problems I face in trying to review research. I know that research is always inherently biased in favour of the prevailing consensus, but this bias occurs so early on in the process that you cannot possibly know that it ever happened. How can you spot the missing paper that might have been published, if the authors had been brave enough to do the study in the first place... but chose not to or didn't get the funding from their own departments? How can you read the paradigm changing paper that was turned down by peer reviewers?

At present, eager post-graduate students with their first research project will be directed to study areas that are unlikely to disturb whichever hypothesis currently holds sway. If they do actually start research into 'uncomfortable' areas, funding will be far more difficult to obtain. If, despite this, they manage to finish a paper, it is far less likely to be published.

You think not...

"According to the founder of Evidence Based Medicine experts are hindering the healthy advancement of science.

"Writing in this week's British Medical Journal (BMJ), Canadian-based researcher, David Sackett, said that he would 'never again lecture, write, or referee anything to do with evidence based clinical practice.'

"Sackett is not doing this because he has ceased to believe in evidence based clinical practice but, as the BMJ comments, because he is worried about the power of experts in stifling new ideas and wants the retirement of experts to be made compulsory.

"Sackett claims that the prestige of experts (including himself) gives their opinions far greater persuasive power than they deserve on scientific grounds alone. 'Whether through deference, fear, or respect, others tend not to challenge them, and progress towards the truth is impaired in the presence of an expert,' he writes.

"He also argues that expert bias against new ideas operates during the review of grant applications and manuscripts. 'Reviewers face the unavoidable temptation to accept or reject new evidence and ideas, not on the basis of scientific merit, but on the extent to which they agree or disagree with the public positions taken by experts on these matters.'"[76]

Chaos theory suggests that exceedingly small effects can have a massive impact in the end. A butterfly flaps its wings in Brazil and causes a massive storm in Australia – that sort of thing.

An idea first thought of several centuries ago:
For want of a nail the shoe was lost.
For want of a shoe the horse was lost.
For want of a horse the rider was lost.
For want of a rider the battle was lost.
For want of a battle the kingdom was lost.
And all for the want of a horseshoe nail.

(Children's nursery rhyme).

If small unconscious effects can massively bias an outcome, then how much more distortion can be created if the entire system is using various mechanisms to actively maintain the status quo. Add into this the intense social pressure that we all feel to fit in with our peer-group, and defer to experts, and you can see why Max Plank observed that 'truth never triumphs.'

I would, perhaps, be somewhat less negative. I do feel that the truth will, even must, eventually triumph – even if it takes several lifetimes to emerge. Because the truth, when it *is* true, is immortal. You cannot kill it, the best you can do is concrete it over. It may lie dormant for years, but given the slightest encouragement it bursts forth again.

When everyone with a vested interest in suppressing the truth has lost the reason to keep on doing so it will be re-discovered. Someone asked me recently, when will the cholesterol hypothesis die? My reply was 'shortly after the last patent on the last cholesterol lowering agent expires.' Once the financial foundations are no longer there, the empire of the cholesterol hypothesis will be swept away by the marauding Goths, Huns and Visigoths. I hope I shall be there to witness it.

However, this perhaps takes me too far away from the point of this section, which is to highlight the extraordinary difficulty of challenging the status quo. Which is pretty much the same thing as the view of the alpha male experts in a given area of medicine. Yes, this is very much a testosterone-driven world.

This is a difficulty further compounded by the fact that the experts have attained the status of demi-gods. Recently, I was reading an article on Daniel Kahneman, Nobel Prize winner in economics. He was discussing the irrationality of the financial system. He made many interesting points. For example:

"The way scientists try to convince people is hopeless because they present evidence, figures, tables, arguments, and so on. But that's not how to convince people. People aren't convinced by arguments, they don't believe conclusions because they believe in the arguments that they read in favour of them. They're convinced because they read or hear the conclusions from people they trust. You trust someone and you believe what they say. That's how ideas are communicated. The arguments come later."

Slightly later on, he talks about his own belief in global warming:

"Why do I believe global warming is happening? The answer isn't that I have gone through all the arguments and analysed the evidence – because I haven't. I believe the experts from the National Academy of Sciences. We all have to rely on experts."

In one breath he states that people aren't convinced by arguments; they're convinced because they read or hear conclusions from people they trust. Then he says that we all have to rely on experts. But he does not link these two thoughts together to ask the obvious question. Just how, exactly, did the experts come to *their* conclusions?

By listening to people they trust? And whom might they be? Other experts, presumably. And how did they come to their conclusions...? By listening to other experts. And how did they come to their conclusions...? Hold on, it seems we are trapped in a loop of self-reinforcing logic. There is no escape.

The alternative is to believe that experts do not listen to people they trust. Instead they scrutinise the evidence, figures, tables and arguments. At which point they come to their conclusions. Conclusions with which we must just agree. In order to go along with this argument, we have to accept that experts are superior to normal people and use only, logic. We the 'lumpenproletariat', however, can merely expect to bumble about, guided by the wise experts, in whom we must trust. These experts are a higher kind of being.

Which leads on to the next question. How does one become an expert in the first place? Is there a secret handshake? Clearly you cannot become an expert by disagreeing with any other experts as they must, by definition, be right. As Kahneman states "*We all have to rely on experts.*" It sure makes life simple. Don't think... obey. '*You there, you epsilon semi-moron with the heart attack – get back in bed... now!*' Sound of bleating in the background. '*All praise the alphas...* '

I do know that the media is completely and utterly in their thrall. Because of my controversial views about heart disease, statins and the like, I am often contacted by journalists. Once I have convinced them that a raised cholesterol does not cause heart disease there is a pause... and I know exactly the question that is coming next...

'Which experts support your point of view?'

Here is an example of an e-mail received from a journalist:

"We have spoken in the past about the cholesterol-heart disease causation question: A book about this issue by Prof Philippe Even has just been published in France, and American guidelines on heart disease treatment which are due out sometime soon, are expected for the first time to move away from an ever-lower cholesterol target.

"NICE is also reviewing its guidelines, and I wondered if you know if anyone has emerged in the UK cardiology hierarchy or broader medical establishment who might raise any question about the cholesterol hypothesis?

"Any suggestions would be very gratefully received."

A journalist

I wrote back

"You may as well expect the enclave in the Vatican to vote for a Jew.
"Sorry, when the dam bursts, all the cardiologists will claim they never believed in the Cholesterol hypothesis. It's all inflammation dontcha know. As for now, first to break ranks gets shot."

Once a journalist asks me for the name of an 'expert' who will support me I know that nothing I have said (or very little), is then going to see the light of day. For they will contact the British Heart Foundation, or Flora (hard to tell the difference nowadays), and ask for the *expert* view on the matter. This, to my utter amazement, is exactly the same view as they have held for the last 20 years. Saturated fat in the diet raises cholesterol levels, raised cholesterol levels causes heart disease... end of discussion. Dr Kendrick is talking nonsense.

They will normally add in a comment such as '*all of the experts agree*', and throw in some barbed comment about my lack of expertise. When faced with a tightly knit bunch of highly decorated experts, most journalists can clearly see which side the bread is buttered – or would that be Flora'd (if that is now a verb).

I have virtually given up explaining to journalists that experts will always hold exactly the same view as each other. If they did not, they would – by definition – no longer be experts. A dissenting expert is a contradiction in terms. You are either with us, or against us. One might as well ask a Manchester City supporter if he knows of any other Manchester City supporters who support Manchester United.

Which of course means that someone like Dr Uffe Ravnskov – a longtime critic of the cholesterol hypothesis – simply cannot be an expert. He has written three books on heart disease and the diet-heart/cholesterol hypothesis. He has published many papers in various journals (and has had far, far more rejected). He has spent 40 years of his life studying heart disease and is both a qualified medical doctor and PhD. But he doesn't hold the mainstream view, and thus he cannot be considered an expert.

In short everything is loaded in favour of the status quo, or the prevailing dogma, or whatever you want to call it. So, it should come as little surprise to find that, when Ionnadis started to look at medical research he found that.

"Moreover, for many current scientific fields, claimed research findings may often be simply accurate measures of the prevailing bias."

J Ionnadis

A view supported from a slightly different angle by Dr Marcia Angell, who was the editor of the *New England Journal of Medicine* for two decades. This was, and remains, the single most powerful and influential medical journal in the world. At least it is, when it comes to citations and impact factor:

"It is simply no longer possible to believe much of the clinical research that is published, or to rely on the judgment of trusted physicians or authoritative medical guidelines. I take no pleasure in this conclusion, which I reached slowly and reluctantly over my two decades as an editor of The New England Journal of Medicine."[77]

Now there's a damning indictment from the editor of the journal with the highest 'impact factor' in medical publishing. If she came to the realisation that published clinical research cannot be believed – what hope is there? She was reviewing, allegedly, the highest quality research papers in the world.

As for the quality of published research itself, here is one of my favourite quotes by Drummond Rennie, at the time the Deputy Editor of the *Journal of the American Medical Association*:

"There seems to be no study too fragmented, no hypothesis too trivial, no literature citation too biased or too egotistical, no design too warped, no methodology too bungled, no presentation of results too inaccurate, too obscure, and too contradictory, no analysis too self serving, no argument too circular, no conclusions too trifling or too unjustified, and no grammar and syntax too offensive for a paper to end up in print."[78]

I would add a caveat to that quote... 'so long as it supports the status quo.'

Of course we have a major problem here. Ionnadis, Angell and Rennie are widely respected 'experts' in medical research, and they are telling us that much, if not most, of the research published is biased, untrustworthy and, quite often, the most complete rubbish. So the other experts must be, it seems, not quite as believable as some would wish.

Where then, does that leave us with regard to Kahneman's statement *"We all have to rely on experts"*? Which experts to believe? Those who tell us that the experts are publishing papers that are biased, untrustworthy, warped and bungled? Or those experts who manage to get those papers published in the first place? Without disappearing into a black hole of circular arguments what can you believe? What is your position?

Skeptical. I hope. But with a few relatively simple rules to follow:

Rule one. Experts are, frankly, no more likely to be right about any given scientific hypothesis than you. But they are much better at marshalling the troops, and their heavy artillery will outgun yours. However, do not be cowed by their, apparent, superior knowledge and intellect. They are like the Wizard of Oz. Look behind the screens, and there is a little old man pulling the levers whilst pretending that he is big and scary.

Rule two: The angrier an expert becomes, the more likely they are to be wrong (when the flak is at its greatest you know you are nearing the target). An angry expert is a wrong expert.

Rule three: When an expert is wrong, he, or she, is far less able to change their mind than you. Because it matters so much more to them than anyone else. Their entire reputation, status, and income, may be built on the hypothesis they now support.

"Nothing is more flatly contradicted by experience than the belief that a man, distinguished in one of the departments of science is more likely to think sensibly about ordinary affairs than anyone else."

Wilfred Trotter

"The most resilient parasite is an idea."

Inception (the film)

CHAPTER SEVEN

Games are played and the players are…

Despite what I have just written about 'experts' being wedded to their 'expert' views, I do not think that there can be any doubt that the single most important reason why medical research is corrupted is money. Money acts like a great tsunami, driving everything before it in one direction, and one direction only, in favour of the pharmaceutical company, which dishes out the moolah.

There are many different ways in which money distorts the world of medical research. We're going to call them "games", although they are anything but fun.

Game 1 – Fund the studies

The first step in the process is that pharmaceutical companies fund and run most of the major clinical studies on drugs, and other interventions.

This is where bias starts, although it is often impossible to spot it. How can you know which important end-points were *not* included in a clinical trial, and why? Why was comparator drug x chosen and not drug y? Why did they choose statistical test z? Why did they exclude patients with heart failure, or diabetes, or decide on combined end-points? There are a myriad ways to bend the results to your will, long before a trial starts.

Here is a 'tip of the iceberg' list published in the *Public Library of Science*, from a talk by Richard Smith (ex-editor of the *BMJ*):[79]

"Examples of Methods for Pharmaceutical Companies to Get the Results They Want from Clinical Trials:

- *Conduct a trial of your drug against a treatment known to be inferior;*

- *Trial your drugs against too low a dose of a competitor drug;*

- *Conduct a trial of your drug against too high a dose of a competitor drug (making your drug seem less toxic);*

- *Conduct trials that are too small to show differences from competitor drugs;*

- *Use multiple endpoints in the trial and select for publication those that give favourable results;*

- *Do multicentre trials and select for publication, results from centres that are favourable;*

- *Conduct subgroup analyses and select for publication those that are favourable;*

- *Present results that are most likely to impress – for example, reduction in relative rather than absolute risk."*

I could add a few hundred more subtle ways than that, but life is too short.

In the early days, a great deal of research was carried out in major teaching universities. Opinion leaders would set up the trials, run the research, and analyse the results. They tended to have a simple agenda. Does this drug work, or not? How touchingly naïve.

By 2005 less than a third of drug related studies were being done in academic units. To quote from an ethics feature in *The Journal of the American Board of Family Medicine*:

"The removal of research from academic centres also gives pharmaceutical companies greater control over the design of studies, analysis of data, and publication of results.

*"The end result: among even the highest quality clinical research the odds are **5.3 times greater** that commercially funded studies will support their sponsor's products than non-commercially funded studies. The authors conclude, 'Readers should carefully evaluate whether conclusions in randomized trials are supported by data.' Careful readers with enough time can sometimes spot discrepancies between data and conclusions in published studies. However, the drug companies typically retain control over the data from their sponsored trials so the **majority of the researchers don't have open access to the results from their own studies." (My emphasis).*[80]

In short, whilst spotting all of the bias in commercially funded studies is impossible, we do know that the combined effect of data manipulation by the industry is to change the odds in their favour by, at least,

530%. 'Yes, ladies and gentlemen, let me introduce the new blood-pressure lowering drug with a whopping 530% bias built in right from the start.'

Although the myriad of manipulations mostly remain hidden, from time to time the distortions can breach the surface, and emerge, blinking into the light, like a giant deep sea animal appearing from the depths. Just to give one example, over the years there have been many, many, statin trials done. They have almost exclusively been funded by the pharmaceutical industry, and they have all managed to prove that statins are beneficial (to some degree or other).

All that is, except one. This study was funded by the US government, and it went by the catchy title of the Antihypertensive and Lipid Lowering Treatment to Prevent Heart Attack Trial (ALLHAT-LLT). And what did this study find?

"Washington, DC – Surprising results of an unblinded but randomized comparison of pravastatin (Pravachol® – Bristol-Myers Squibb) vs 'usual care' in patients with hypertension and moderate hypercholesterolemia enrolled in the Antihypertensive and Lipid Lowering Treatment to Prevent Heart Attack Trial (ALLHAT-LLT) show that pravastatin did not significantly reduce either all-cause mortality or fatal or nonfatal coronary heart disease (CHD) in these patients."[81]

Well, there you go. This study found that statins provided absolutely no benefit at all. Of course the findings were immediately attacked, and rubbished. My favourite argument came from an American cardiologist. In an editorial accompanying the publication, Dr Richard C. Pasternak (Massachusetts General Hospital, Harvard Medical School) writes:

"Physicians might be tempted to conclude that this large study demonstrates that statins do not work; however, it is well known that they do."[82]

Perhaps he needs to be introduced to Karl Popper and his concept of refutation. It runs something like this. If your hypothesis is that '*All swans are white,*' the fact of finding another white swan may increase the propensity of your hypothesis by a small amount. However, if you find one black swan, your hypothesis is dead. Unless, of course, you are happy to simply flat out ignore the finding, as per Pasternak.

In fact, I think that Richard Pasternak's statement can be altered very slightly to the following – without losing the slightest meaning. '*Physicians might be tempted to pay attention to evidence, but they should* *not. I shall tell them what to think instead. Do not trouble your pretty little heads with such trivial nonsense as evidence. Listen to **me,** the mighty Richard Pasternak.'*

So, on one hand, we have 30 or so pharmaceutical company funded studies demonstrating the inarguable benefits of statins. On the other hand, we have one independent study demonstrating that statins don't work. Which study should you believe? Well, I know which of the 31 studies I consider to be the black swan and the effect it has on the hypothesis.

Interestingly, when he wrote that highly scientific refutation of the ALLHAT trial, Dr Richard C. Pasternak was a cardiologist at Massachusetts General Hospital. I note that a few years later he become Vice President, Head Global Scientific Affairs and Scientific Leadership at Merck. Do Merck make statins and other lipid lowering agents... well, by golly, I believe that they do. What an amazing coincidence. Astonishing, how on earth do you think such a thing could possibly have happened?

Forgetting Dr Pasternack for a moment, it is clear that pharmaceutical funding of clinical trials creates bias... At least 530% bias – whatever exactly that means, but it sounds like a big number to me. However, the inherent bias doesn't stop here by any means. In reality it doesn't actually start here. It begins far, far, earlier.

Game 2 – Create a disease to be treated

It starts with the creation of diseases. There can be few things worse for a pharmaceutical company than having a product, without a disease to treat. The best thing to do in this situation, obviously, is to create a disease to match your product. Here's Wikipedia on Female Sexual Arousal Disorder:

"Female sexual arousal disorder (FSAD), commonly referred to as Candace syndrome, is a disorder characterized by a persistent or recurrent inability to attain sexual arousal or to maintain arousal until the completion of a sexual activity. The diagnosis can also refer to an inadequate lubrication-swelling response normally present during arousal and sexual activity. The condition should be distinguished from a general loss of interest in sexual activity and from other sexual dysfunctions, such as the orgasmic disorder (anorgasmia) and hypoactive sexual desire disorder, which is characterized as a lack or absence of sexual fantasies and desire for sexual activity for some period of time.

"Although female sexual dysfunction is currently a contested diagnostic, pharmaceutical companies are beginning to promote products to treat FSD [Wiki mysteriously drops the "arousal"] often involving low doses of testosterone."

146

OK, they are having a bit of trouble convincing people that FSAD is a disease. But other 'diseases' can be created. For instance Syndrome X:

"Most people may not have heard of metabolic syndrome, but that is likely to change. Once known mysteriously as Syndrome X, the condition, a precursor to heart disease and type 2 diabetes, is about to be transformed into a household name by the US pharmaceutical industry and its partners in the medical profession. A society dedicated to addressing the condition has been organized, a journal has been started, and an education campaign launched. Patients are already being tested for metabolic syndrome. As the trade publication Pharmaceutical Executive *said in its January 2004 issue:* **'A new disease is being born.'**"[83]

In fact, Syndrome X was strangled at birth. And perhaps for a very simple reason. Metabolic syndrome included: raised blood pressure, low HDL (good) cholesterol levels, insulin resistance/raised blood sugar, obesity, and many other 'abnormalities.'

If you were to cure syndrome X, a vast chunk of the pharmaceutical market would disappear in front of your very eyes. No need for blood pressure medication, anti-diabetic medication, HDL raising agents, obesity medications, and so and so forth. We hear little of syndrome X these days. Nearly made a horrible mistake there guys.

However, not all attempts at creating diseases are unsuccessful. Far from it. One area where new diseases are plucked out of the air, at will, is in psychiatry. In 1952 the first edition of the book 'Diagnostic and Statistical Manual of Mental Disorders' (DSM-I) came out. It listed 106 mental diseases (including homosexuality). We now have 374 mental disorders (DSM-IV). So, there are now 268 new forms of mental illness. Each one with a drug attached – virtually.

To quote from Gøtzsche's book again, talking about the DSM categories:

*"According to Frances (Allen), new diagnoses are as dangerous as new drugs: 'We have remarkably casual procedures for defining the nature of conditions, yet they can lead to tens of millions being treated with drugs they may not need, and that may harm them. Drug regulatory agencies should therefore not only evaluate new drugs but should also oversee how new '**diseases**' are being created. The confusion and incompetence is so great that the DSM-IV cannot even define what a mental disorder is.'"[84]*

By the way Frances Allen, quoted above, chaired the committee that created DSM-IV. He now believes that responsibility for the defining psychiatric conditions should be removed from the American Psychiatry Association. The chances of this happening are beyond fat.

He has further warned that DSM-V will almost certainly unleash multiple new false epidemics, not only because of industry money, but also because researchers push for greater recognition of their pet conditions. In his view, DSM-IV created three false epidemics because the diagnostic criteria were set far too wide. In particular he cites: ADHD, autism and childhood bipolar disorder.

I confidently predict that despite warning from the likes of Frances Allen, DSM-V will continue where DSM-IV left off. More diseases created, more new and expensive drugs found to treat them, more money to be made. Yes, creating diseases is a highly profitable game. Just look at raised cholesterol. Billions upon billions.

If creating diseases seems like too much effort, you can simply adjust the criteria for existing illness. By widening the diagnostic boundaries you can ensure that almost everyone is ill. In depression for example (according to DMS-IV) you can now be diagnosed as being depressed if:

You had little interest or pleasure in doing things for more than half of the days over the past two weeks, plus one additional symptom, such as:

- Trouble falling asleep;

- Poor appetite or overeating;

- Being so fidgety or restless that you have been moving around a lot more than usual.

Well, that's me depressed for starters.

Narrowing the boundaries of 'normal' is a technique used in many different areas of medicine. When I graduated in medicine, a high cholesterol was 7.5 mmol/L. Then it became 6.5, then 5.5, now it is 5. Or 4, if you have had a heart attack or stroke. In the latest US guidelines 'optimal' cholesterol level for healthy people is 4.4 mmol/L (In US units this is 170 mg/dl).

By driving the definition of high cholesterol ever downwards, we have reached the point where more than 85% of people now have a 'high' cholesterol level, which needs to be lowered. This is fine so long as you do not question the inherent nonsense that the vast majority of the population can possibly have a dangerously high level of something. Ever come across the concept of 'average' guys?

'You are a slow learner, Winston.'

'How can I help it? How can I help but see what is in front of my eyes? Two and two are four.'

'Sometimes, Winston. Sometimes they are five. Sometimes they are three. Sometimes they are all of them at once. You must try harder. It is not easy to become sane.'

Exactly the same process is happening with blood pressure, blood sugar levels, weight, HDL etc. The boundaries in all of these areas tighten and tighten. Even if your cholesterol level is found to be 'optimal', once you feed the other risk factors into the latest risk calculators for cardiovascular disease the chances are virtually 100% that something will be 'abnormal'. At which point you will be informed that you will need to take a drug of some sort – for the rest of your life. Kerching!

This has become so completely ridiculous that, according to the latest American guidelines, if you are a man, by the time you are 63 and you have no risk factors whatsoever for cardiovascular disease: perfect weight; no diabetes; cholesterol optimal; blood pressure super-optimal... You still need to go onto a statin.[85]

Which means that we have reached that situation where you have no risk factors for a disease; but you still need to take a drug to prevent that very disease? Logic has left this land, to be replaced by the low humming sound of money being pumped directly into pharmaceutical company bank balances.

In reality, you don't actually need to use the risk calculator. You already know your official 'statin by date.' Once you have reached this age, just head down to the pharmacy and pop some money in the statin dispenser. For women your statin-by-date is a bit later than mine.

If you are female and utterly and completely healthy (according to the risk calculator) your 'statin-by-date' is 70. (However, your chances of being completely healthy are... zero.). An interesting twist on Logan's Run. Another interesting twist is that the patient leaflets for statins caution against their use by the over 70s, so women should go on them and immediately come off them as they blow out their 70 candles. This is probably because low cholesterol in elderly people is seriously bad for longevity.

Running close behind cholesterol, the definition of type 2 diabetes has continued to tighten inexorably, with lower and lower blood sugar levels being considered dangerously high. This was entirely predictable.

What was also entirely predictable was the creation of a condition known as 'pre-diabetes'.

As with 'pre-hypertension', if you have 'pre-diabetes,' whilst you are not yet diabetic you are clearly heading that way. In the UK it is estimated that 7,000,000 adults have pre-diabetes – that's around 25% of the adult population.

By now you should have a pretty good idea of where this particular story ends:

"The diabetes drug Actos (pioglitazone), which increases insulin sensitivity, appears to dramatically lower diabetes risk in people with prediabetes, according to a new study. People with prediabetes who took the drug had a 72% reduction in diabetes risk, compared to patients who did not take it, researchers report.

"They estimate that one case of diabetes could be prevented if 18 high-risk people were treated with the drug for a year. The study appears in the March 24 issue of The New England Journal of Medicine. The findings suggest that millions of people at high risk for diabetes may benefit from taking Actos..."[86]

Of course, Actos happens to be a drug that works in exactly the same way as Avandia. This drug was, as you may remember, withdrawn due to increasing the overall death rate. More recently, Takeda was fined $6,000,000,000 for hiding data on Actos increasing the risk of stomach and pancreatic cancer. A mere $6 billion.

Yes, this story will end with millions and millions and millions more people taking drugs to treat their 'pre-diabetes'. It hardly needs to be said that the financial pressure for this to happen is gigantic. Just imagine the market size. It would make any pharmaceutical company executive drool at the prospect.

If there are 7,000,000 pre-diabetics in the UK, there must be 40,000,000 in the US, and probably another 200,000,000 world-wide (in countries rich enough to matter to the industry). We are talking a quarter of a billion people here. If you managed to get even one tenth of them onto Actos that represents a market of 25,000,000 people.

Each Actos pill costs at least $1.50 (lowest end estimate).

If we do a rough calculation:

25,000,000 x $1.50 x 365(days) = $13,687,500,000 (Nearly $14 billion/year).

Oh my Lord, be still my beating heart, and wipe that drool from my face.

With that type of money on offer you can see why it will not be long before various drugs will be approved for use in pre-diabetes.

Depressingly, about a week after writing that sentence, someone sent me a news story from Australia announcing that pharmacists would "become fat cops". A leaked document from the Department of Health revealed plans for pharmacists to check the weight, blood pressure, blood sugar and cholesterol of all Australians once a year. The powers-that-be reckon **up to 60 per cent of people with pre-diabetes could be prevented from progressing to the disease as a result of these checks.** [87]

That was February 2014. In June, England followed by declaring that "One in three adults in England has pre-diabetes."[88]

Apart from creating diseases, and inexorably narrowing the boundaries of health, another great way to expand the market is talk up the dangers of existing and well established diseases.

Game 3 – Turn a non-illness into a crisis e.g. Tamiflu

As a GP, I was taught that flu was basically a self-limiting illness. Patients who caught it should stay at home, deal with their symptoms and not 'bother' the doctor. A few elderly or very young patients could develop serious complications, and might need to be treated for secondary infections and suchlike. Other than that, there was not much to do.

Then, suddenly, flu became a deadly killing monster that must be treated with drugs. I was working in local surgeries and OOH (Out of Hours) during the winter of 2009/10 when the *great swine-flu pandemic of terror*' erupted.

We were swamped. The demand for vaccination for children went through the roof. At the same time it was decreed that anyone with swine-flu had to be treated with Tamiflu (made by Roche).

It was total chaos. Special help lines were set up to decide who should have Tamiflu – manned by people who had been, almost literally, dragged off the streets. After an in-depth intensive two week training course, these newly qualified doctors suddenly had the magical power to diagnose swine-flu, over the phone, without doing any tests, or seeing the patient... (don't get me started, at least three patients almost certainly died in our local area due to being diagnosed with swine-flu over the phone, when they had something else).

Doctors' surgeries nearly snapped under the strain. It was like something out of a science fiction movie when the great mutant virus hits. The end result of the *'great swine-flu pandemic of terror'* was that... about the same number of people as normal died of flu that year (probably fewer). It turned out to be hyped up nonsense, as I bloody told anyone who would listen at the time.[89]

However, it was also extremely profitable for Roche, the makers of Tamiflu who, in an act of great generosity agreed to sell the UK Government hundreds of millions of pounds worth of Tamiflu. Nice of them, don't you think?

It amused me to note that, by the end of the *'great swine-flu pandemic of terror'* Tamiflu was getting handed out like sweeties, as the tablets started to reach their sell by date. Waste not, want not.

Of course Tamiflu is exceedingly effective and wonderful, and saved thousands of lives. The evidence supporting its use was rigorous and water-tight... Ho... ho. Not.

"The British Medical Journal (BMJ) has alleged that pharmaceutical giant Roche is deliberately hiding clinical trial data about the efficacy of oseltamivir (Tamiflu) in patients with influenza. The journal says global stockpiling and routine use of the drug are not supported by solid evidence and alleges that Roche concealed neurological and psychiatric adverse events associated with the neuraminidase inhibitor drug.

"In an open letter from Fiona Godlee, MD, editor-in-chief of BMJ, to Professor John Bell, FRS, HonFREng, PMedSci, Regius Professor of Medicine at Oxford University in the United Kingdom and a Roche board member, published online December 2012, Dr Godlee reminds Bell of concerns that were initially voiced in 2009 about the reliability of Tamiflu research.

"At that time, BMJ published an updated Cochrane review of neuraminidase inhibitors in healthy adults. That study 'took the view that, since eight of the 10 [randomized controlled trials] on which effectiveness claims were based, were never published, and because the only two that had been published were funded by Roche and authored by Roche employees and Roche-paid external experts, the evidence could not be relied upon,' Dr Godlee writes."[90]

In short, there is little or no evidence that Tamiflu does any good at all. And the data that it may do harm has never been published. In fact, it is being deliberately withheld from the UK government by that super-ethical company called Roche.

You may be aware of the Tamiflu battle that is still rumbling. Despite repeated requests, Roche simply refuse to release critical data. I wonder why?

Could it be that Roche knows that Tamiflu either doesn't work very well (if at all), or causes lots of adverse effects... or both? I put my money on both.

However, to return to the main theme here. Flu used to be seen as a relatively mild disease – apart from the dangers to those in a small high risk group. However, when a drug appeared to treat flu, and I use the word 'treat' in a very loose fashion, we suddenly find that flu has become a dangerous killer.

Was this whole nonsense primarily hyped up by the 'experts' in infectious diseases? To be more specific, was it hyped by experts with close financial ties to companies making anti-flu products?

"Academics with competing interests were nearly six times as likely as those without industry links (p=0.009) to predict a higher risk to the public from the pandemic than was given by official agencies... Academics who promoted the use of antiviral drugs in the UK media during the 2009-10 HIN1 flu pandemic were eight times as likely to have links with the drug industry as quoted academics who didn't comment on their use."[91]

Financial considerations led to the experts with major conflicts of interest hyping up the dangers of swine flu, to ensure that massively expensive and useless drugs are prescribed, which may have damaged millions of people...

1. I solemnly pledge to consecrate my life to the service of humanity;

2. I will give to my teachers the respect and gratitude that is their due;

3. I will practice my profession with conscience and dignity;

4. The health of my patient will be my first consideration;

5. I will respect the secrets that are confided in me, even after the patient has died;

6. I will maintain by all the means in my power, the honour and the noble traditions of the medical profession;

7. My colleagues will be my sisters and brothers;

8. I will not permit considerations of age, disease or disability, creed, ethnic origin, gender, nationality, political affiliation, race, sexual orientation, social standing or any other factor to intervene between my duty and my patient;

9. I will maintain the utmost respect for human life;

10. I will not use my medical knowledge to violate human rights and civil liberties, even under threat;

11. I make these promises solemnly, freely and upon my honour.

I think points four and six of the Geneva Declaration may be worth reviewing in this case. This is just one story of many.

Diseases created, the boundaries of health narrowed, and the health impact of diseases hyped. All of this market manipulation often kicks in long before any drug appears on the horizon. So that, by the time a drug is actually launched, the market is crying out for it.

This all means that the 530% of detectable bias to be found in clinical trials, may sit on top of a far larger mountain of market manipulation that most people are completely unaware of.

However, even after the market has been prepared, and the studies designed and manipulated, the bias continues using a very simple and straightforward technique. Positive studies get published; negative studies are buried... literally in some cases.

Game 4 – Let there only be good news

*"Publication bias, however, remains the most devastating potential bias. The reasons for the non-publication of studies vary. The authors of a small study with unexciting results may have little interest or motivation in getting the study published. More pernicious is the situation where a substantial study is not published—and even purposefully suppressed—because the authors or **funders do not like the look of the results**."[92] (my emphasis).*

Yes, if a pharmaceutical company does not like the look of the results, the trial results do not see the light of day. It is pretty easy to work out that if you only publish positive studies and hide the negative, the bias effectively becomes infinite. See what happens to your calculator if you try to divide any number by zero.

The effects of this particular problem do not represent some theoretical statistical game with your calculator, however. These unpublished data can, and do, kill. The commentary that follows comes from the *Canadian Medical Association Journal (CMAJ).*

The authors looked at how GlaxoSmithKline's (GSK) suppressed negative findings about the effects on suicide and depression caused by their drug, paroxetine. The fact that such negative studies even existed only came to light because GSK were dragged into court in the USA, where they were forced to release internal documents:

"An internal document advised staff at the international drug giant Glaxo-SmithKline (GSK) to withhold clinical trial findings in 1998 that indicated the antidepressant paroxetine (Paxil in North America and Seroxat in the UK) had no beneficial effect in treating adolescents.

"Paroxetine is 1 of 6 drugs in the class of selective serotonin reuptake inhibitors (SSRIs) that Britain and the US have since banned for pediatric use because of increased risk of suicide. On Feb. 2, Health Canada issued a public warning that the pediatric use of 7 antidepressants — paroxetine, bupropion (Wellbutrin), citalopram (Celexa), fluvoxamine (Luvox), mirtazapine (Remeron), sertraline (Zoloft) and venlafaxine (Effexor) — should proceed only after consultation with the treating physician 'to confirm that the benefits of the drug still outweigh its potential risks.'

"The GSK internal document obtained by CMAJ offers a glimpse into the inner workings of a drug giant. Entitled "Seroxat/Paxil Adolescent Depression: Position piece on the phase III clinical studies," the confidential document was prepared by the Central Medical Affairs team (CMAt), a division of SmithKline Beecham (which subsequently merged with Glaxo Wellcome to form GSK).

"The document provides guidance on how to manage the results of 2 clinical trials conducted into the efficacy of paroxetine (Seroxat). Given that the clinical trials results were, according to the document, 'insufficiently robust' to support an application to regulatory authorities for a label change approving Seroxat for use in pediatric depression, CMAt recommended the firm 'effectively manage the dissemination of these data in order to minimize any potential negative commercial impact.'"[93]

I love phrases like *"effectively manage the dissemination of these data in order to minimize any potential negative commercial impact."* I savour the bland, corporate-speak. The utter lack of emotion and meaning. I prefer to express what they did in another way. *'Bury the data, then lie, so we can all get rich. Even though we know our drug is causing children to commit suicide.'* Because that, ladies and gentlemen, is exactly and precisely what they did.

Does that sound a tad harsh? Well, GSK were eventually fined $3,000,000,000 (three *billion* dollars) in 2012 for burying trial data, whilst continuing to promote the use of paroxetine in children. So the courts seem to share my view that GSK did not act according to the highest ethical standards.

A three billion dollar fine may seem massive. In reality, it represents about one quarter of the total sales of paroxetine over the years.[94] I suppose GSK considers a fine of this size to be simply the cost of doing business. Write it off against tax, and it doesn't look so bad. The shareholders will still get a good bonus – as will the CEO.

Following cases like the one described above, and others too numerous to mention, action was supposed to have been taken to ensure that negative data could not simply be buried. Although, for all the effect it had, it may be more accurate to say that a great deal of hot air was expended into the atmosphere debating the issue.

Having said this, it was decreed in 2005 by the International Committee of Medical Journal Editors that they would never again publish a clinical trial unless it had been properly registered first. This was supposed to ensure that you couldn't just pretend a negative study had never taken place before dropping the data down a mineshaft... in Cheshire (UK), if you wanted to know. Of course it hasn't really worked out like that:

Here is Ben Goldacre talking about this issue, seven years after the problem with trial registration had been 'solved.'

"Many people think this problem has already been solved. The medical journals said they weren't going to publish trials that hadn't been registered and there were steps by the U.S. government to require it...

"But unfortunately there was no routine public audit and when one was finally done, many years after this rule came into play, we discovered that academic journal editors hadn't kept that promise.

"[A study published in a major journal] found that half of all the trials published in the top ten journals in the big five fields of medicine weren't properly registered and [many] weren't registered at all—and that's only the ones that we know about."[95]

Once again, this problem is almost certainly worse than Ben Goldacre makes out. Because you still don't know how many unregistered trials were buried. And these may well be the most important. Negative data are often more powerful than positive.

In short, despite apparent agreement to stop it happening, trials are not being registered, and negative data are still not being published. If you want more in-depth analysis of how widespread data manipulation can be, I suggest you read Ben Goldacre's '*Bad Pharma.*' In addition you may want to read '*Deadly medicines and organised crime – how big pharma corrupted healthcare,*' by Peter Gøtzsche.

Game 5 – Be the hand that feeds

Right from the very start of drug development, the industry and high ranking doctors a.k.a. 'experts' work hand in glove. Experts in the world of medical research are often called Key Opinion Leaders (KOLs), for the simple reason that they lead medical opinion. Once again, long before the clinical studies on drugs have been organised, the industry is already pumping money into KOLs.

To quote Marcia Angell once more:

"No one knows the total amount provided by drug companies to physicians, but I estimate from the annual reports of the top 9 U.S.-based drug companies that it comes to tens of billions of dollars a year in North America alone. By such means, the pharmaceutical industry has gained enormous control over how doctors evaluate and use its own products. Its extensive ties to physicians, particularly senior faculty at prestigious medical schools, affect the results of research, the way medicine is practiced, and even the definition of what constitutes a disease."[96]

Opinion leaders have always been of great value to the pharmaceutical industry. There are obvious advantages to the industry in nurturing sympathetic opinion leaders. Primarily because they add scientific and ethical credibility. For those of you reading this who are KOLs or who work for the pharmaceutical industry, I ask you to read to the end of this chapter. Yes there may be some unpalatable information, but that is good. I just think that the public should know about the process so that they can decide for themselves as to whether they follow guidelines or if they want to have a sensible conversation with their doctors about, for example, screening or taking a statin.

If Pfizer says something good about their own drug then this will be seen as advertising, pure and simple. If Professor Albert Hasswinder: MBBA, FRCS, PhD, DipMedSci, president of the European Society of Medicine, editor of the Royal Journal of the British Society of Medicine says it... well, it carries that much greater weight. (For reasons of libel, this is of course a completely made up person).

Not only this, but Key Opinion Leaders can also help enormously in ensuring that drug trials are published in highly respected journals such as the *BMJ*, the *NEJM* and *The Lancet*, which is critically important to success.

None of this comes cheap. KOLs are not cheap – and why should they be. These are very bright people who have worked their butts off. Over time, however, they moved from 'not cheap' to eye-wateringly expensive.

I know of one Nobel Prize winner who wanted, and got, $50,000 to give a one hour presentation at a major meeting. Other top dogs attending international conferences give several different lectures a day – sometimes literally running from room to room because they are massively overbooked.

In the past, in the evenings, at such meetings, pharmaceutical companies then conduct 'expert' advisory boards. Strangely, these board meetings can appear almost indistinguishable from expensive meals in Michelin starred restaurants. With all this money pouring in, even a fairly low ranking Key Opinion Leader can command honoraria (a posh word for great wodges of money) of tens of thousands of dollars per day during international meetings.

Thankfully, a lot of the worst excesses are in the past. There is the Sunshine Act in the US which requires full disclosure of all payments by companies to doctors. Tighter rules and regulations are in place to control ghost writing, hiding clinical trial protocols and just refusing to publish negative data. So, there is hope for improvement. However, it does need to be borne in mind that almost every single drug on the market today was developed, marketed and sold using techniques that were very, very dodgy.

At one time Key Opinion Leaders became so important that an entire industry sprang up around how best to manage them. Software programmes have been developed to identify those with the greatest global reach and the ability to influence guidelines, and Governments.

Here is an advert from a company which does exactly that. It is called KOL L.L.C:

"As our name implies, we are a company devoted to providing Key Opinion Leader software and Key Opinion Leader Management services for pharmaceutical, biotechnology and device companies. We have invented two world-class proprietary web-based applications for managing and developing relationships with KOLs (some have described them as 'knowledge management systems'). More importantly, because we have actual real-world experience from working in the Pharma industry we provide unparalleled service and consulting. We have held positions in medical/scientific affairs, medical science liaisons, medical education, drug information, sales training, strategic marketing, product management and field sales.

"The principals in KOL, L.L.C. have deep experience in cardiology, anti-infective, pain management, diabetes, gastroenterology, urology, women's health and central nervous system products. As such, we have developed personal relationships with many KOLs.

"We are 'The Key to Opinion Leader Development.™'"[97]

Here is a section from an industry report called 'KOL management solutions.'

*"According to Dan Mintze, senior director, heartbeat experts, "The management of KOLs needs to be broader than identifying, segmenting, influence mapping and working with clinicians in order for products to gain clinical approval. Rather a comprehensive KOL solution which includes the identification and appropriate engagement of KOLs who impact market access decisions e.g. KOLs who serve as Government or payer advisory board members (see figure 3) should be adopted." Such pharma-KOL engagement will lead to the development of value messages that can help pharma to access the market faster, gain quicker product adoption, and **increase bottom line performance**." (My emphasis).[98]*

Most Key Opinion Leaders remain utterly convinced that they are in charge of what happens in their therapeutic areas. They believe that they are unbiased, and are merely providing high quality consultancy advice. They think that they are the organ grinders and the pharmaceutical industry the monkeys who dance to their tune. In truth, as the above advertorials make clear, KOLs are viewed by the industry as just another resource which can be used to **increase bottom line performance** (marketing speak for 'making loads of money by selling more drugs'). (My emphasis again).

Just to give one example to demonstrate the power of Key Opinion Leaders, it is salutary to look at cholesterol lowering. There is a committee called the National Cholesterol Education Programme (NCEP). The NCEP sits within the *National Heart, Lung, and Blood Institute (NHLBI)*, which in turn is part of the National Institutes of Health:

"The National Institutes of Health (NIH), a part of the U.S. Department of Health and Human Services, is the nation's medical research agency—making important discoveries that improve health and save lives."

Following this so far? Good, then I hope that you can see that the NCEP is, essentially, a US Government funded and sanctioned advisory group. They produce guidelines on lowering cholesterol levels, what the levels should be lowered to, and suchlike. Their guidelines also carry the force of law in the US. In that, if you don't follow them, you can be successfully sued for medical malpractice.

In addition, such is the power and influence of the US, particularly in the world of medicine, that the NCEP guidelines are usually, if not inevitably, taken up around the globe – with some local adaptations. Indeed, this is exactly what did happen.

If NCEP members decide that the cholesterol treatment targets should be lowered then this has enormous financial implications. From a commercial perspective the decision to lower the target cholesterol levels resulted in tens of **billions** of additional profit, per year, for pharmaceutical companies who made statins. (Less so now, as most statins are off-patent).

So, the experts involved really should have had no financial connections with the pharmaceutical industry. Should they not?

Well, here is a financial disclosure statement regarding NCEP members:

ATP III UPDATE 2004: FINANCIAL DISCLOSURE

Dr Cleeman: (Chairman) has no financial relationships to disclose.

*Dr Grundy: has received honoraria from **Merck, Pfizer**, Sankyo, **Bayer, Merck/Schering-Plough, Kos**, Abbott, **Bristol-Myers Squibb**, and **AstraZeneca**; he has received research grants from **Merck**, Abbott, and Glaxo Smith Kline.*

*Dr Bairey Merz: has received lecture honoraria from **Pfizer, Merck**, and **Kos**; she has served as a consultant for **Pfizer, Bayer**, and EHC (Merck); she has received unrestricted institutional grants for Continuing Medical Education from **Pfizer**, Procter & Gamble, **Novartis**, Wyeth, **AstraZeneca**, and **Bristol-Myers Squibb** Medical Imaging; she has received a research grant from **Merck**; she has stock in Boston Scientific, IVAX, Eli Lilly, Medtronic, Johnson & Johnson, SCIPIE Insurance, ATS Medical, and Biosite.*

*Dr Brewer: has received honoraria from **AstraZeneca, Pfizer**, Lipid Sciences, **Merck, Merck/Schering-Plough**, Fournier, Tularik, Esperion, and **Novartis**; he has served as a consultant for **AstraZeneca, Pfizer**, Lipid Sciences, **Merck, Merck/Schering-Plough**, Fournier, Tularik, Sankyo, and **Novartis**.*

*Dr Clark: has received honoraria for educational presentations from Abbott, **AstraZeneca, Bristol-Myers Squibb, Merck**, and **Pfizer**; he has received grant/research support from Abbott, **AstraZeneca, Bristol-Myers Squibb, Merck**, and **Pfizer**.*

*Dr Hunninghake: has received honoraria for consulting and speakers bureau from **AstraZeneca, Merck, Merck/Schering-Plough**, and **Pfizer**, and for consulting from **Kos**; he has received research grants from **AstraZeneca, Bristol-Myers Squibb, Kos, Merck, Merck/Schering-Plough, Novartis**, and **Pfizer**.*

> *Dr Pasternak: has served as a speaker for **Pfizer, Merck, Merck/Schering-Plough**, Takeda, **Kos, BMS-Sanofi**, and **Novartis**; he has served as a consultant for **Merck, Merck/Schering-Plough**, Sanofi, **Pfizer** Health Solutions, Johnson & Johnson-Merck, and **AstraZeneca**.*
>
> *Dr Smith: has received institutional research support from **Merck**; he has stock in Medtronic and Johnson & Johnson.*
>
> *Dr Stone: has received honoraria for educational lectures from Abbott, **AstraZeneca, Bristol-Myers Squibb, Kos, Merck, Merck/Schering-Plough, Novartis, Pfizer**, Reliant, and Sankyo; he has served as a consultant for Abbott, **Merck, Merck/Schering-Plough, Pfizer**, and Reliant.[99]*

Those companies marked in bold sell (or at the time sold) statins and/or other cholesterol lowering medications. The others, of course, were just innocent bystanders. A mere 8 members (the chairman was employed by the NIH and was not allowed close ties with industry), had almost 70 direct financial conflicts of interest with companies who made cholesterol lowering agents.

I would like to imagine what would happen if the Supreme Court made a decision on a commercial issue of major worldwide importance, and then revealed that they had 70 direct financial conflicts of interest. Or eight politicians, or eight journalists. The outcry would be heard across Galaxies. Doctors, however, are obviously beyond any possibility of corruption. Gasp, choke, thud.

Did the money make a difference to their decisions? For an insight into this, I am grateful to a Dr John Kassirer who put together a compare and contrast presentation. He looked at the NCEP guideline recommendations for primary prevention of heart disease. He then compared them with the recommendations made by the University of British Columbia (UBC), which is part of the worldwide Cochrane collaboration.

The Cochrane collaboration accepts no sponsorship from industry – at all. Not for itself, or its researchers. (Yet, strangely, they are still considered experts. Did they not know that unconflicted researchers are not truly expert)?

Unfortunately, Kassirer was not comparing identical reviews here. In mitigation, I have not found a single example where that would be possible. However, the reviews are based on very similar evidence, and they were done within a year or so of each other. The NCEP reviewed five statin trials, and the UBC reviewed five statin trials. Three trials were exactly the same, two were different – though closely related.

The recommendations from the two groups were, as follows:

NEW NCEP GUIDELINES JULY '04

NCEP: Reviewed these studies:

PROSPER
ALLHAT-LLT
ASCOT-LLA
PROVE IT-TIMI 22
HPS

Recommendation:

Aggressive LDL lowering for high risk patients [primary prevention] with lifestyle changes and *statins.*

THERAPEUTICS INITIATIVE U.B.C. 2005

UBC: Reviewed these studies:
PROSPER
ALLHAT-LLT
ASCOT-LLA
AFCAPS
WOSCOPS

Conclusion:

Statins have not been shown to provide an overall health benefit in primary prevention trials.

The NCEP group of experts, with very strong financial ties to companies marketing statins, concluded that statins should be used 'aggressively' in primary prevention. The Cochrane Collaboration group of experts, with no financial ties to industry, concluded that statins should not be used in primary prevention. What a remarkable coincidence that is... or perhaps not.

Now for any KOLs and Pharmaceutical folks still reading at this point – and I hope some of you are – I think I should make it clear that not all, and possibly a minority of, this collaboration between the industry and KOLs is corrupt, biased, prejudiced or negative in any way. At one time I worked with opinion leaders to develop educational programmes for the use of warfarin in atrial fibrillation to prevent strokes. This has become a highly beneficial treatment that has delayed (even prevented) many thousands of disabling and fatal strokes. Without the knowledge, connections, influence, and sheer hard work of many KOLs, this may never have happened at all.

Many opinion leaders are also highly ethical. They are motivated by a desire to develop and introduce best treatments, and the money they are paid is consistent with the value that they bring to the table. They are exceedingly bright and hardworking, and why shouldn't they be paid the going rate?

Also, just because someone is paid to say something, this does not mean they don't believe what they are saying. It can become easy to fall into the so-called 'motive fallacy', which is the notion that if you have some particular interest (financial or otherwise) in holding an opinion, this must automatically render it untrustworthy. Most doctors, for example, really do believe that statins are wonderful. You don't need to pay them anything to say this... unfortunately.

However, some opinion leaders do flip over to the dark side. I know of some 'experts' who, in the past, if they were going to a conference overseas, would speak on behalf of five different companies and charge each of those companies a separate first class air fare to get there – in cash. Usually, they demanded the money up front for first class tickets, not only for themselves but for their entire family, who never actually left home. Just where did that money go? Hey, swimming pools cost a lot of money, dontcha know.

Thankfully, a significant amount of this behaviour is historical. Over time, the excesses just became too great, and there was something of a backlash. Here is a salutary tale from the USA, discussing Dr Fred Goodwin, a psychiatrist in the USA. He was in the sights of Senator Grassley who was, and remains, on a crusade against the pharmaceutical industry:

"Two days after lashing into Fred Goodwin, who hosts 'The Infinite Mind' on National Public Radio, US Senator Chuck Grassley is now investigating Best Practice, a pharmaceutical consulting firm that Goodwin helped establish in the late '90's. Among the many services that have been offered by the firm – marketing consultations to drugmakers and the 'dissemination of new off-label information.'

"Doctors can prescribe a drug to treat an illness even if the FDA has not approved that use, but promotion of off-label activity is a big no-no. So in a letter

sent today to Roger Meyer, who heads the firm, Grassley wants to know more about Best Practice's questionable practices. The Senator notes that the claims can be found on older versions of the firm's web site.

"How did Grassley find Best Practice? By investigating Goodwin, who we wrote about earlier. Last March, an episode of his program, 'The Infinite Mind,' which is heard on 300 NPR stations, featured three experts who discussed the controversial link between antidepressants and suicide. And all four, including Goodwin, declared that worries about the drugs have been overblown.

"As it turns out, Goodwin also had undisclosed ties to drugmakers. Since 2000, for instance, Glaxo paid Goodwin more than $1.2 million in speaking fees and over $100,000 in expenses. And Glaxo markets the Paxil antidepressant, which UK regulators determined that the drugmaker had been aware since 1998 that its pill was associated with a higher risk of suicidal behavior in adolescents. NPR is embarrassed and angry by all this and yanked the program from its satellite service."[100]

The key phrase in this was case is that the NPR was embarrassed and angry about Goodwin's actions. So much so, that they yanked his program from its satellite service. At which point Fred Goodwin (what is it about that name) was no longer an asset for Glaxo. He instantly became a liability. You are not much use to the industry once your credibility has evaporated.

Another very high profile doctor, and his entire unit, also came under fire at about the same time. Eric Topol became 'famous' for attacking a drug called Vioxx, which was developed for use in arthritis. He was lauded by many for bravely taking on the giant pharmaceutical company Merck. But...

A 2004 article by Bethany McLean, in *Fortune* magazine, questioned Topol's own potential financial conflicts of interest. She reported that Topol served as a scientific advisor to a hedge fund which profited substantially by short selling Merck stock. The very Merck stock that plummeted when Topol raised concerns about Vioxx. Topol denied giving the hedge fund advance information, severed his ties to industry and donated all such income directly to charity. How kind of him. In a 2005 *JAMA* commentary, Topol stressed that *"no true conflict of interest existed in this case."*[10]

"In November 2005, Topol was subpoenaed in a class action lawsuit against Merck. He testified that Vioxx posed an "extraordinary risk", and that Raymond Gilmartin, former chief executive officer of Merck, had contacted the head of the Cleveland Clinic board to complain about Topol's work on Vioxx.

"Two days afterward, Topol was informed that the position as chief academic officer at the Cleveland Clinic had been abolished, and he was removed as provost of the Cleveland Clinic Lerner College of Medicine, which he had founded. The Clinic described the timing as coincidental. The New York Times described Topol's demotion as part of an 'unusually public dispute' between Topol and the Cleveland Clinic's chief executive, Delos Cosgrove, and stated that Topol's criticism of Merck had focused scrutiny and criticism on the Clinic's deep and longstanding ties to the pharmaceutical and medical-device industries."[102]

So, apparently, we have an opinion leader working hand in glove with a hedge fund. He is intimately involved in a court case against Vioxx, and, after his public criticism of the drug, Merck stock just happened to plummet. At the same time, the hedge fund he was working with made millions short-selling Merck stock. Yet Topol states, hand on heart, that *"no true conflict of interest existed in this case"*?

Ladies and gentlemen of the jury. If that does not constitute a conflict of interest 'true' or otherwise – then what on Earth does? I do not believe it is humanly possible to be more conflicted than that. And why would a physician 'associate' himself with the investment industry in the first place? The words *'to earn vast sums of money'* spring to mind...

Game 6 – Forget or hide having been 'fed'

The whole area of doctors working closely with the industry comes under the banner of conflict of interest. At this point I must disclose that it is not just KOLs who are accused of this. I have been accused of having conflicts of interest. I wrote a comment in a doctor's discussion forum about statin side-effects, and that they were far more common than most people thought. Another doctor claimed that as I wrote *The Great Cholesterol Con*, I should declare my conflicts in this area, as I could just be trying to sell more books.

I told him to get stuffed. In my view a conflict of interest is that you are being paid money by someone else. I have been a critic of statins since they first came out, and no-one has ever paid me anything to state this. So I am not conflicted in that I am saying exactly what I have always said – in books and out.

Whilst it is not possible to read anyone's mind to know if they are saying things they believe, or are being paid to say, it is possible to strip things down to basics. In the past, too many highly influential doctors were paid very large sums of money by pharmaceutical companies. It is beyond the slightest doubt that this has created significant bias in favour of those companies and has resulted in products being promoted, and approved, that perhaps should never have reached the market.

Everyone knows that this is a major problem. But nothing has really been done. If you are caught out, what happens? Why, almost exactly nothing. You can just mutter *'I didn't realise this was a conflict of interest,'* and that's usually about the extent of any punishment. For example, a few doctors were 'named and shamed' by the *Journal of the American Medical Association*, when someone pointed out that a number of authors of their original paper might just have slipped up in declaring their conflicts:

Unreported Financial Disclosures in: 'Association of LDL Cholesterol, Non-HDL Cholesterol, and Apolipoprotein B Levels With Risk of Cardiovascular Events Among Patients Treated With Statins: A Meta-analysis.'
*... the following disclosures should have been reported: Dr Mora reports receipt of travel accommodations/meeting expenses from **Pfizer**; Dr Durrington reports provision of consulting services to **Hoffman-La Roche**, delivering lectures or serving on the speakers bureau for **Pfizer**, and receipt of royalties from **Hodder Arnold Health Press**; Dr Hitman reports receipt of lecture fees and travel expenses from **Pfizer**, provision of consulting services on advisory panels to **GlaxoSmithKline, Merck Sharp & Dohme, Eli Lilly**, and **Novo Nordisk**, receipt of a grant from **Eli Lilly**, and delivering lectures or serving on the speakers bureau for **GlaxoSmithKline, Takeda**, and **Merck Sharp & Dohme**; Dr Welch reports receipt of a grant, consulting fees, travel support, payment for writing or manuscript review, and provision of writing assistance, medicines, equipment, or administrative support from **Pfizer**, and provision of consultancy services to **Edwards, MAP**, and **NuPathe**; Dr Demicco reports having stock/stock options with **Pfizer**; Dr Clearfield reports provision of consulting services on advisory committees to **Merck Sharp & Dohme** and **AstraZeneca**; Dr Tonkin reports provision of consulting services to **Pfizer**, delivering lectures or serving on the speakers bureau for **Novartis and Roche**, and having stock/stock options with **CSL** and **Sonic Health Care**; and Dr Ridker reports board membership with **Merck Sharp & Dohme** and receipt of a grant or pending grant to his institution from **Amgen**.[103]*

Not a bad little list. As you can see, Dr Ridker had actual *board membership* with Merck Sharp and Dohme, a company that has made billions from selling statins. Here is he is authoring a paper on the benefit of statins, and he simply *forgot* about the fact the he was sitting on the board of MSD (Or maybe he didn't)? As for the others, well, they're also busy people, things must have just slipped their minds, such as 33 separate financial conflicts of interest.

For this terrible crime against the integrity of medical science none of them can ever again do medical research, or author a medical paper. Cue, mad, cackling laughter. Or sound of head beating repeatedly against wall. As you may expect, absolutely nothing happened at all, apart from the quiet publication of the above statement in the *Journal of the American Medical Association (JAMA)*. 'Nothing to see here, move along.'

A few years ago, aware that things had possibly gone too far, and that the credibility of the medical profession was looking a bit tarnished, a number of doctors made a move which has made things worse, and more opaque. They appeared to take a step back from the industry, and financial conflicts of interest... At least on paper they did.

Following Topol's lead, an increasing number of KOLs started to make public announcements that they would not take any money directly from industry, and they would donate any money they earned from working with the industry to charity.

For example, after Eric Topol 'left' the Cleveland Clinic, Dr Steven Nissen took over much of his work. Here is a disclosure statement by Dr Steven Nissen. I think it is a complete belter. Is there any company that he doesn't work with?

Dr Steven Nissen
Medical Director
Cleveland Clinic Cardiovascular Coordinating Center

Dr Nissen has received grant/research support from AstraZeneca Pharmaceuticals, Atherogenics; Eli Lilly and Co., Lipid Sciences, Pfizer Labs, Sankyo Pharma, sanofi-aventis, and Takeda Pharmaceuticals North America **with all reimbursement directed to the Cleveland Clinic Cardiovascular Coordinating Center**; *and has been a consultant for Abbott Laboratories, AstraZeneca Pharmaceuticals, Atherogenics, Bayer Corp., Eli Lilly and Co., Forbes Medi-tech, GlaxoSmithKline Pharmaceuticals, Haptogard, Hoffman-LaRoche, Isis Pharmaceuticals, Kemia, KOS Pharmaceuticals, Kowa Optimed, Lipid Sciences, Merck/Schering Plough, Novartis Pharmaceuticals Corp.,*

---

*Novo-Nordisk, Pfizer Labs, Protevia, Roche Pharmaceuticals, Sankyo Pharma, sanofi-aventis, Takeda Pharmaceuticals North America, Vasogenix, Vascular Biogenics, Viron Therapeutics, and Wyeth Pharmaceuticals, **all fees are paid directly to charity with no reimbursement paid to Dr Nissen**; and has served on the speakers' bureaus of AstraZeneca Pharmaceuticals and Pfizer Labs, **all fees are paid directly to charity with no reimbursement paid to Dr Nissen.***

So, Nissen works tirelessly on behalf of 30 impoverished pharmaceutical companies, and he gets paid nothing at all for doing so? And expects nothing for so doing? The pharmaceutical companies, in turn, expect nothing from him, or his institution. And his institution does not mind the fact that he must spend a great deal of time doing voluntary work on behalf of starving pharmaceutical companies?

Nissen is not alone in this opaque new world of unpaid charity work for the pharmaceutical industry. The whole *'giving any earnings to charity'* thing has spread. In the UK, we have the Clinical Trial Service Unit (CTSU) at Oxford. This unit, like the Cleveland Clinic, runs massive clinical studies on behalf of the pharmaceutical industry.

Of course this is very good news for the pharmaceutical companies, in that the CTSU is a part of Oxford University. This ensures that any research that emanates from it sounds exceedingly academic and prestigious, and also untainted by grubby pharmaceutical interests. It is certainly more impressive sounding than calling it a commercial clinical trials unit which is, in reality, exactly what it is.

Here is a part of the CTSU guidelines:

Guidelines for CTSU staff with respect to honoraria and any other payments offered and share ownership:
d: If an honorarium is declined, the intended CTSU recipient can still mention that a corresponding amount might be donated to a specific charity.

What does this mean? Why would you do work for the pharmaceutical industry then have it all paid into a charity? Well, it might be that all the people working at the Cleveland Clinic and the CTSU are either exceedingly rich, or the most ethically and morally principled people on Earth. Or perhaps something else is going on here.

Here is a quote from an investigative journalist on the matter:

"I guess if I had any advice for reporters, I would say, ask your local university if they've set up any associated [non-profit organizations]; many universities have an associated charity or foundation through which they solicit donations from corporate sponsors to support medical research. Find out about who those corporate sponsors are. Unfortunately, many universities set up these associated charities and foundations in such a way that they don't have to disclose much publicly – ask about that, you know, try to push."[104]

Push away, but you won't get very far. What I know for certain is that the CTSU has received hundreds of millions in funding from the pharmaceutical industry.[105] Professor Sir Rory Collins is a director of this unit, and he is paid by the CTSU. Despite this, he feels able to state that he has absolutely no financial conflicts of interest, because he is not paid 'directly' by the industry.[106]

Anyway, it would appear that we have now reached the situation as follows:

- If a pharmaceutical company slips the dosh into your back pocket, you are conflicted, but if you forget to declare it, don't worry – nothing happens. If you do declare it, nothing much happens either.

- If a pharmaceutical company pays the dosh to the CTSU, or the Cleveland Clinic, or some other such organisation, which then pays the dosh to you, this means that you are not conflicted in any way. You do not even, it seems, have to make a conflict of interest statement.

- You can also ask for any payment you might receive to be paid to a 'charity'. (We'll look at this one next). These charities are strangely difficult to pin down, and may be directly linked to the institution that you work for, and may even be run by your wife (yes, you know whom I am talking about).

Is this right, or wrong? I know what I think. I think that we need to get a grip on this problem and not allow opinion leaders to decide whether or not they believe they have a conflict of interest, before deciding whether or not they can be bothered declaring it. What I would like to do is follow the money trail. It cannot be that difficult. In fact it has been made easier in the US with the Sunshine Act ensuring that any payment of more than $10 must be declared. (But only if it comes from the industry).

169

Of course it is not just the opinion leaders and experts who receive money or gifts, or free education meetings in fancy hotels. Humble GPs also receive money and gifts. They are far smaller. Although, perhaps, far more cost effective.

"The evidence is clear: gifts, even small ones, change behaviour... Social science research ... shows that a gift of any size imposes on the recipient a sense of indebtedness. This need for reciprocity is a deep-seated human reaction. It creates in the recipient, whether consciously or not, a sense of obligation to repay favors, gifts, invitations, etc. Research shows that it takes extraordinarily little to bias an individual's interpretation and processing of information. Such bias is both subtle and unintentional."[107]

Game 7 – Give to charity

So far, we have seen that pharmaceutical companies may control, and manipulate the data from clinical trials. They also pay very large sums of money to key opinion leaders who run the trials, to ensure that:

"... pharma-KOL engagement will lead to the development of value messages that can help pharma to access the market faster, gain quicker product adoption, and increase bottom line performance."

Billions are also spent on sales forces who set up 'educational' meetings, bombard doctors with carefully crafted messages, and shower them with gifts. Less so in the UK, the EU and the USA over the last few years, as more and more rules now govern such interactions.

Things, however, do not stop here, far from it. In the US, vast sums of money are spent on direct to consumer advertising. This is not allowed in Europe, but it does not stop the pharmaceutical industry from accessing the public in a variety of different ways.

One way is by giving large sums of money to 'charities' such as Heart UK, or the BHF (British Heart Foundation), or Alzheimer's Research. A closely related tactic is to fund patient advocacy groups like the MS society.

The first question to ask yourself here is very simple. Why would a pharmaceutical company give money to charities and patient advocacy groups? Why indeed. To quote from a magazine called *Pharmaceutical Executive*:

"Product managers see advocacy groups as allies to help advance brand objectives, like increasing disease awareness, building demand for new treatments and helping facilitate FDA clearance of their drug."[108]

'Building demand for new treatments'... I wonder what that could possibly mean? Is that the same as increasing bottom line performance, or selling more drugs? Hmmm, let me think about that, for at least an entire nanosecond

Of course, helping to push a drug onto the market may be no bad thing if the drug is of real benefit. However, the simple fact is that pharmaceutical companies do not spend money on any activity before someone has made the case that they can be assured of significant return on investment a.k.a. selling more drugs.

No, they do not fund health 'charities' and patient advocacy groups out of the goodness of their hearts. They do this in order to increase market size and profit – pure and simple. They know the power of patient groups in lobbying politicians. They are ideally placed to get various heart rending stories published in newspapers. *'My son was refused new cancer drug and is going to die...'* That sort of thing.

Dr Barbara Mintzes, a Canadian researcher who has investigated this issue points out that:

"A consumer group funded by telephone companies would not be trusted to judge the best mobile phone package, nor to be a public advocate on telecommunications policy. Is health less important?"

Just to give you some idea of the scale of funding. Here is a list of the corporate partners of the Alzheimer's Society in the UK. Not all of them are pharmaceutical companies, several are.

CORPORATE PARTNERS WITH THE ALZEIMERS SOCIETY[109]

Adecco; Advantage; Ageas Insurance; Airbus; Ametis Furniture (South West); Anchor Care Homes; Ascot Underwriters; Athompson; Barchester Healthcare; Barclays HR; Barratt Homes (Bristol); Baxter; Begbies Traynor; Beta; (The) Bingo Association; Boundary Mill Colne; Boundary Mill Store Grantham; Bristan Group; Bunzl; Bupa; Capita; Certeco; Charity Flowers; Circle Partnership; Deans Garden Centre; DLA Piper Leeds; DLA Piper Liverpool; Dulux Decorator Centres; Dundas and Wilson; Ellis Whittam; ES Pipelines; Field Fisher Waterhouse ; GCA (United Utilities); Geldards LLP; Gelder Group; Hays Recruitment; Herbert Smith; HSBC; Insolvency Company; Jehu Group; LABC; (The) Lawyer Awards; Levicks Accountants; Lilly UK; Lloyds Banking Group; MCI (Petersfield); MGM Advantage; MHS Homes; Moneysupermarket.com;

Some of these companies might be providing funding through a sense of public good. Others, such as Bupa, Barratt Homes, Saga Homecare, Sunrise Senior Living etc. etc. are directly involved in building nursing care homes for dementia patients, looking after them, and charging them large sums of money for so doing. I don't see, for example, Mothercare in this list, or Pampers nappies. I wonder why.

The first question to ask, about charities associated with healthcare, is: what are they, exactly? In what way are they charitable? Many charities are very clearly in the business of doing good work for starving children in Africa, and suchlike e.g. Oxfam.

But when you get to healthcare, the 'charitable' aims can become significantly less clear. Heart UK, for example, is 'The Cholesterol Charity.' This organisation was presumably set up to help poor starving cholesterol molecules.

Actually, here is a statement of aims, values, and marketing waffle. It has a vision, a mission and values, no less:

HEART UK is the Nation's cholesterol charity.

Vision: To prevent avoidable and early deaths caused by high cholesterol.

Mission: To provide support and prevent high cholesterol driven conditions through our services.

In 5 years time (2016), we want the majority of UK adults to know their cholesterol levels, understand the impact and to be taking any necessary action.

Values: To place the needs of patients and their families at the centre of our work.

In order to assist them in this valuable work, they have enlisted the help of the following organisations. (Those who sell cholesterol lowering products/services, or are involved in marketing such products, are marked in bold):

172

> *ABPI Scottish Cardio Vascular Industry Group; Alere; Alpro; Astra-Zeneca UK Limited; Bayer Schering Pharma; Boehringer-Ingelheim; Bristol Myers Squibb; Cereal Partners UK (Shredded Wheat); Complete Medical Communications (Takeda); Fresenius Medical Care (UK) Limited; Genzyme; Kellogg's (Optivita); Kowa Pharmaceutical Europe Co Limited; LINC Medical Systems Limited; Lloyds Pharmacy Limited; Lodestone Patient Care; Merck Pharmaceuticals; Merck Sharp & Dohme Limited; Pfizer Limited; Point of Care Services Limited; Premier Foods; Randox Laboratories Limited; Sanofi-Aventis Ltd; Schering Plough Ltd; Shellfish Association of Great Britain and SHELLFISH; Solvay Health Care; Takeda; Welch's; Unilever (Flora); Unimedic.*

Oops, sorry, they are all in bold, aren't they? I wonder how that happened?

Apparently, if you work with Heart UK, and pay to use their logo on your product then there is – according to the makers of Shredded Wheat – '80% added trust' in the eyes of the consumer. This type of added trust has, according to the Welch's (who make antioxidant grape juice), greatly increased the sales of their product.

The only bit of this statement you really need to remember is this: *"greatly increased the sales of their product."*

You can find this out from looking at the corporate charity connection video on their website – if you would ever wish to do such a thing. And here was me thinking these companies worked with Heart UK out of the kindness of their HEART UKs. Nothing to do with increased sales, or anything as grubbily commercial as that. Well, maybe not.

As it turns out, charities can be organisations that are funded by Merck, and Pfizer and Astra Zeneca and Unilever. Then cardiologists can do work for Heart UK, and be paid by them for such work, yet have no financial conflicts of interest to declare vis a vis Merck, Pfizer, Astra Zeneca, Unilever and suchlike... Discuss (shouldn't take that long to discuss I would imagine).

If we look at another health charity, it becomes clear that commercial sponsorship stretches as far as the eye can see. I found this list on page one million, subsection three trillion of the Diabetes UK website. Or, to put it another way, this charity doesn't exactly trumpet their corporate sponsorship.

They also, very coyly, don't say: "Here is a long list of companies who have paid us great wodges of money." They call such things corporate 'acknowledgments.' You know, you really should call a spade, a spade.

The commercial interests of most of these sponsors here are obvious. Abbott, Pfizer and Lilly all have diabetes pharmaceutical products to sell. Flora is obviously trying to sell Flora margarine to everyone without functioning taste buds, especially patients with diabetes, who need to avoid those terrible saturated fats.

However, some associations seem be less obvious. For example, Kodak. Why would they sponsor Diabetes UK? They make cameras and photocopiers and printers and suchlike, don't they? What interest could they possibly have in diabetes? Well, let me think... Do they, perchance, make blood sugar monitors? Why, of course, they do.

You mean Kodak are not just handing over money to Diabetes UK for the good of society? They want some influence in the market. No, surely not. Next you will be telling me that Disneyland wasn't just set up as a charity to allow children from around the world to have lovely holidays.

Game 8 – Write government policy

This is the last game to share with you and it's a good'un. The pharmaceutical industry has now managed to achieve something it could surely only have dreamed of. It is hiring pharmaceutical company lobbyists to create NHS policy documents:

I wrote a blog about it:

"The pharmaceutical industry now controls NHS policy – hoorah."[110]

Here is the offending headline from the Guardian newspaper: "NHS hires drugmaker-funded lobbyist."

As the secondary headlines say:

"Conflict of interest concerns as Specialised Healthcare Alliance (SHCA), funded by pharmaceutical companies, advises NHS England.

174

"A lobbying organisation with links to some of the world's biggest pharmaceutical companies and medical equipment firms has been asked by NHS bosses to write a report that could influence health policy, it has been reported."

It seems lobbying is now *'so five minutes ago.'* Who needs a lobbyist when this organisation, the Specialised Healthcare Alliance (SHCA), which is entirely bought and paid for by the pharmaceutical industry, has been commissioned to write a report on funding specialised services for the NHS. Services worth £13,000,000,000-£20,000,000,000. That's £13-20 billion per year.

The article does point out, though, that we are misguided to think that this could in any way be an issue for concern. John Murray, the director of the SHCA, a lobbyist, and author of the report, has made it clear that:

"...there was no link between his lobbying business and the SHCA other than providing secretariat services and said the SHCA 'never takes a position on particular products or treatments in any of its activities.'"

John (Pinocchio) Murray's nose is now in the Guinness Book of Records for being the longest nose ever recorded on a human being, at seven point three miles. He is a lobbyist, paid for by pharmaceutical companies, and his organisation never takes a position on particular products... hahahahahahahahahaha! Well then, sack him immediately for being useless... sack him for failing to do what he is handsomely paid to do.

The final part of this newspaper report, which I savoured, is the following:

"James Palmer, clinical director of specialised services at NHS England, said he was aware of Murray's role as a lobbyist but 'there are no opportunities for lobbying in the process of forming clinical policy.'"

This, of course, is true. There are no opportunities for lobbying in this particular process of forming clinical policy. Once a lobbyist starts to write clinical policy they have moved well past the annoying requirement to lobby anyone. For the lobbyist has now managed to become the very person that they should be paid to lobby in the first place.

Instead of trying to influence someone who may not listen to him, he can just talk to himself... Imagine that this short section of imagined dialogue is like Smeagol talking to Gollum in Lord of the Rings (Smeagol and Gollum are, of course the same person):

John Murray: *We must put the following phrase into the report, my precious. A* **"clear commitment"** *to* **"disinvest in interventions that have lower impact for patients"** *in favour of* **"new services or innovations".**

John Murray: *But why would you like me to put this in the report, won't this harm the hobbits? Hobbits have been kind to me... yes they have.*

John Murray: *I need it in the report you fool. I represent precious pharmaceutical companies that are bringing new products onto the market. We needs to ensure that there will be plenty of money to pay for them. So they must stop paying for stupid old fashioned treatments... yes, they must, foolish Hobbits.*

John Murray: *But won't the kind Hobbits be worried this will just look like lobbying.*

John Murray: *Don't be so stupid. How can the nasty Hobbits accuse me of lobbying? I am their friend, and I am trying to help them... yes I am.. Yes John Murray likes the friendly Hobbits. John Murray want to help the Hobbits, yes he does.*

John Murray: *You are so clever Smeagol, our master will be pleased...*

Duchess: "You're thinking about something, my dear, and that makes you forget to talk. I can't tell you just now what the moral of that is, but I shall remember it in a bit."

"Perhaps it hasn't one," Alice ventured to remark.

"Tut, tut, child!" said the Duchess. "Everything's got a moral, if only you can find it."

Where we are now

I'll leave it to the *BMJ* to sum up here:

"The power of drug companies to buy influence over every key group in health care—doctors, charities, patient groups, journalists, politicians—has clearly shocked a UK parliamentary committee. It should shock us all. Can we console ourselves that companies' lavish spending on research and marketing, which far outstrips spending on independent research and drug information, leads to truly innovative treatments? No, says the committee's report. Can we rely on regulatory bodies to keep the industry in check? No, again."[111]

In his book, Professor Gøtzsche states:

"Bribery is routine and involves large amounts of money. Almost every type of person who can affect the interests of the industry has been bribed: doctors, hospital administrators, cabinet ministers, health inspectors, customs officials and

political parties. In Latin America, posts as minsters of health are avidly sought, as these ministers are invariably rich with wealth coming from the drug industry.

"In the beginning of this chapter, I asked the question whether we are seeing a lone bad apple now and then, or whether pretty much the whole basket is rotten. What we are seeing now is organised crime in an industry that is completely rotten."[112]

Gulp. In short, my fears of an effective totalitarian regime are not some whacko conspiracy theory about the future. They are fears about what is happening right now. At the risk of over-relying on one article I shall quote again from Iona Heath:

"Reviewing George Orwell's 1984 in 1949, the American critic Lionel Trilling wrote: 'He is saying, indeed, something no less comprehensive than this: that Russia, with its idealistic social revolution now developed into a police state, is but the image of the impending future and that the ultimate threat to human freedom may well come from a similar and even more massive development of the social idealism of our democratic culture.

"Arguably, the current ascendancy of medical technology is just such a manifestation of social idealism. War is peace: ignorance is strength: freedom is slavery – and now we have the latest example Orwellian doublespeak... Health is disease.'

"Trilling continues: 'The essential point of 1984 is just this, the danger of the ultimate and absolute power which the mind can develop when it frees itself from conditions, from the bondage of things and history.'

"The sorts of measurement that underpin the imperatives of contemporary medicine – blood pressure, serum cholesterol, bone density, PHQ9 depression score, body mass index, estimated glomerular filtration rate, just to mention a few – are all held to be universally applicable whatever the circumstance of the individual life to which they are applied. They are in Trilling's words 'freed from condition' and therefore dangerous."

Written in relatively calm academic language what is being said can often sound less worrying than it should be. What Iona Heath is saying should chill us all to our core. She is explaining that we truly are heading for an increasingly repressive Orwellian state. As always this will be hidden under the guise of a beneficial *'Big Brother'* Government protecting the people from health dangers. At the same time ensuring the silence of dangerous reactionaries. Like me, for example.

The simple fact is that over the last 50 years or so, a gigantic interconnected system has been painstakingly constructed. One that is perfectly designed to promote an ever increasing use of drugs, medical devices, and any other form of medical intervention that can make money.

This machine grinds into action long before most people are even remotely aware that a drug even exists. Not infrequently, diseases are created, or adapted, to match up with the drugs that are coming along. Annoyingly trivial diseases can be turned from something mild into life threatening monsters, and so it goes.

Later on, once the marketing strategy has been established, the companies will set up a study in order to demonstrate that their new product provides 'unique' benefits. After thinking about how to set up various end-points, and carefully choosing comparator drugs, and doses, they start the clinical trial, having already identified the key opinion leaders they want to 'run' it.

Once completed, such studies will almost inevitably produce some positive result or other. (If not, hire the gravediggers, and start again). At which point beaming opinion leaders will be lined up to announce their findings at an international medical conference, during which there will be a blaze of publicity.

Medical journalists, usually paid to attend the conference, will be fed carefully crafted PR press releases. The PR message will be taken, pretty much verbatim, and fired out to media outlets throughout the world where they will reappear on the front pages... effectively unchanged.

"'Journals have devolved into information laundering operations for the pharmaceutical industry', wrote Richard Horton, editor of The Lancet, in March 2004. In the same year, Marcia Angell, former editor of the New England Journal of Medicine, lambasted the industry for becoming 'primarily a marketing machine' and co-opting 'every institution that might stand in its way.'

"Jerry Kassirer, another former editor of the New England Journal of Medicine, argues that the industry has deflected the moral compasses of many physicians, and the editors of PLoS Medicine have declared that they will not become 'part of the cycle of dependency ...between journals and the pharmaceutical industry.'"[113]

The journal will then be paid vast sums of money by the pharmaceutical company to produce tens of thousands of re-prints (A few glossy pages containing the clinical study, with the journal title in bold). These re-prints are provided to drug 'reps' to wave in front of doctors. They will be used alongside 'detail-aids' written in order to convince doctors of the benefits of this new wonder drug.

In parallel, the pharmaceutical company will be working with the patient groups and charities that they run (sorry support), in order to create pressure on health authorities and politicians to press for the use of their new drug. Celebrities will be pushed in front of cameras to talk about why they think this drug is so wonderful.

The end game is where opinion leaders who 'ran' the original study are elected to sit on the guideline committees that decide which drugs should be used for condition X. Lo and behold, the drug ends up in the guidelines, which means that doctors will *have* to use said drug. No choice. If you dare disagree with the outputs of these KOLs, you risk being disciplined by the medical authorities. In the US, you can end up in jail (or gaol), if you diverge from guidelines.

As you can see, I hope, the manipulation of the markets created by money happens on such a vast scale that it effectively becomes invisible. When it comes to bias, you are looking for a bit of cheating on the playing field. You didn't realise that the pharmaceutical companies invented the game, built the playing field, wrote the rules, and pay for the officials to make the decisions.

Who is there to stand up to this massively powerful machine?

Whom can you trust?

I wanted to make it exceedingly clear that the question 'whom can you trust' becomes harder and harder to answer when: '*medical technological industries, medical research and regulatory bodies, clinical practice, payment systems, guideline production and national healthcare systems*' are inextricably linked. To this list I would add: governments, healthcare charities and patient support groups.

Journalists... journalists as mentioned before, are supposed to dig out the truth. If not, what is the point of them? However, apart from being bullied into submission, there are other reasons why it is difficult to blame the journalists for their apparent passivity in this area.

They are fed a line and they repeat it – they would be brave not to do so. If they question the official propaganda then they are up against a Key Opinion Leader who will completely baffle them with medical statistics. It is a brave man who dares to take on a medical expert in their own lair. You fear looking foolish, and you also fear that you will say something utterly stupid because you don't really know the area in any great depth. Which means that journalists toe the party line.

So whom can you actually believe, now that I have ruled out almost everyone? Unfortunately, I do not have any certain answers. I can hardly ask you to trust me. As P.G. Wodehouse once said *'when an Englishman says 'trust me' it is time to start counting the spoons.'* Well, I am actually a Scotsman, but the same rule applies. The least trustworthy person is usually the one who announces *'you can trust me on this.'*

There is one ray of light, however. I think you *can* trust the data themselves. However critical I become, however despondent, I do not think that researchers actually falsify the data. Yes, it does occasionally happen, but not often enough to corrupt the entire medical research database beyond all possibility of redemption... I hope (If this is not true, let's hand over the keys, give up and go home).

Of course, studies that are negative are still not published (which is a massive problem) and that is not always the pharmaceutical companies fault – journals don't much like publishing negative data. Studies going in the wrong direction may be stopped, and buried, and end-points can be changed half way through clinical trials. Yes, the data are manipulated and twisted and mangled beyond recognition for publication purposes. But you can usually, with sufficient time and effort, and understanding, pull out most of the real facts and figures and reconstruct much of what was actually found.

Remember that Professor Michel De Lorgeril was able to deconstruct the JUPITER data to find that there were 12 deaths in the placebo arm and 12 deaths in the statin arm? Professor Michel De Lorgeril is someone you can trust. He searches for the truth, and finds it.

As does Dr Uffe Ravnskov, Prof John Anderson, and the unmatchable Prof Paul Rosch. Not forgetting to mention Prof Peter Gøtzsche, Barry Groves (sadly deceased), Dr John Briffa, Gary Taubes, Dr Michel Anchors, and Dr John Ionnadis, and Iona Heath, and others who are far too numerous to mention.

What do these people have in common?

1. They have absolutely no connection whatsoever with the pharmaceutical industry, or any other commercial organisations.

2. They are sceptics who refuse to just accept current dogma – about anything. This is because they know one, very absolutely critical thing. Just because almost everyone says a thing is true – this does not make it true.

Some of those I have mentioned might be wrong about what they believe. I do not agree with Dr Uffe Ravsnkov's ideas about the true causes of heart disease, and he does not agree with mine. But I know, beyond a shadow of doubt that he thinks what he thinks – because he believes it to be true. Not because everyone else says it is true, or because he is being paid to say it.

Thank God that he, and his like, exist. They are the beacons of truth shining out amongst the fog of manipulation and prevarication. When you meet someone searching for the truth you pretty much know when you meet the real deal. They are the people I turn to when I want to know what is real, and what is false.

And what can you, gentle reader, do about the effects that the distorting mirror of money has on medical research? By which I mean, can you spot the distortions, and then make decisions about the data – and whether or not you should pay attention to it?

I wish I had an answer to this. But I don't. Not really. I can only give you some general principles that I use.

1. If there are large sums of money being made from selling a drug then it is absolutely 100% certain that there will be significant bias in the direction of the drug, in all research and publications.

2. Look for the people out there who have a completely different viewpoint from the mainstream. Decide whether or not they sound sensible, and look at the facts and data they present. Does it seem robust? If they pass these basic tests read what they have to say e.g. Ravnskov on the cholesterol hypothesis, Gøtzsche on breast cancer screening, Groves, Briffa and Taubes on weight loss. Lorin on Alzheimer's, Graveline on statins and Alderman on salt. At the very least you should find it interesting, and you will often gain a completely different insight into an area you may have thought was signed, sealed and delivered.

3. Trust yourself to understand what is being said. If you cannot, it is not you – it is them.

4. If you cannot understand what is being said, it is most likely deliberate.

5. Be sceptical.

CHAPTER EIGHT

Doctors can seriously damage your health

For many years I have studied the history of medicine and the ideas that have come and gone. It is easy to look back and laugh at hypotheses that were clearly nonsensical. Here is a little ditty from the eighteenth century lauding the benefits of the tobacco enema.

Tobacco glyster, breath and bleed.
Keep warm and rub till you succeed.
And spare no pains for what you do;
May one day be repaid to you.

Dr Houlston (24 September 1774)

What is that all about, exactly? Well, it was known that tobacco had stimulant properties. If someone was close to death, or even apparently dead through drowning, or suchlike, conventional wisdom was that you could save their life by blowing tobacco smoke up their rectum with a pair of bellows. So strong was this belief that hundreds of set of bellows were hung up around the Thames to revive those who had fallen in and drowned.

The hell with CPR, just blow smoke up someone's backside, that'll do the trick. How idiotic does this now sound? Pretty idiotic I would think. However, very intelligent people believed it was true. Doctors thought it to be true... Not, of course, that I would necessarily confuse doctors with intelligent people.

Sadly, each generation easily convinces itself that such arrant nonsense has become a thing of that past. *'Today, Mr Einstein, we live in a new scientific and enlightened age where only the truest truths, supported by prime quality scientific evidence, are accepted as fact. We can readily sift scientific truth from nonsense.'*

183

I thought I would just slip in the name of Albert Einstein. He was one of the most scathing critics of Wegener's hypothesis on tectonic plate movement. I believe that he called it utter nonsense. Not that I hold anything against Einstein. It just proves that even the most ferociously intelligent people can get things horribly wrong.

You may think it is all very well ridiculing those in past generations who could not understand concepts that an average five year old takes for granted today e.g. the Earth orbits around the sun and not, I repeat, not the other way around.

However, the point here is not ridicule, at least not entirely. It is my attempt to highlight the errant patterns behind thinking that went horribly wrong, especially medical thinking. My hope is that, if we can spot patterns of flawed thinking, this may help to identify some of the errors that we are living with today.

Of course, this is clearly not easy, nor can it ever be 100% accurate. I am a great fan of Karl Popper who believed that predicting the future was impossible. Primarily due to the fact that we can only know a thing once we know it – and we cannot know what we don't know – by definition – until we know it. (Shortest critique of 'The Poverty of Historicism' ever – I claim my prize).

However, just because logic states that it is impossible to know the things that are wrong in advance of them being proven to be wrong, I believe that certain forms of thinking and action do exist that make things far more likely to be wrong, and to later be found to be wrong. When we see three things happening, then alarm bells should start to ring loudly.

They are, in no particular order of importance:

- The need to do something/anything;

- Grabbing the simple/easy hypothesis too early;

- Being so certain your hypothesis is correct you don't do any study to prove that it is beneficial – you just get on with it.

One of my core philosophies is *'Don't just do something, stand there.'* However, a significant majority of the medical profession appears overwhelmed with the need to rush around doing things, no matter what. I sometimes liken them to dog owners who jump into the ocean to save their dogs from drowning, even when they cannot themselves swim. They drown; the dog swims ashore, then gazes curiously around wondering where the hell their owner went.

184

Maybe not the perfect analogy, but I know that few of us are capable of standing back when someone else gets into trouble. The need to do something, anything, is a very powerful human response. It is the old 'baby down the well' syndrome. We strain every sinew, bankrupt the entire community, long after there is any possibility of saving the baby.

Anyone standing around who made a statement. *'There is a very high probability that the baby is already dead, this all seems a complete waste of time and effort, we should just give up and go down the pub,'* would probably be hounded out of town. Giving up is not allowed, you *cannot* give up. Those who spend 72 hours without sleep, digging through rock to get the baby with their bare hands will be seen as plucky heroes. They did everything they humanly could.

The simple fact is that, in order to help others, most people believe that taking action, any action, is a far better option than doing nothing – almost no matter what the chance of success may be. This is an incredibly powerful driver of human behaviour. As a social animal I think it is hard-wired into our brains to help others, and there is little we can do about it. Not that I think we should do anything much about it.

Except, of course, when the irresistible need to do something results in harm rather than benefit.

How bed rest killed

An almost perfect example of this would be the belief in strict bed rest following a heart attack. This was first proposed by John Herrick in his seminal paper on heart attacks/myocardial infarction.

Prior to 1912 no-one had ever fully described a myocardial infarction. Which made this a landmark paper in the history of medical research. Whether or not the first ever heart attack actually occurred in 1912 is a moot point. Frankly, I very much doubt it. Moving on from that issue for the moment, here are some sections from a report on a talk by Dr Braunwald on the deadly consequences of Herrick's first paper.

"In 1912, Dr James Herrick (1861–1954) of Chicago published in JAMA 'Clinical features of sudden obstruction of the coronary arteries.' In that article, he stated, 'The importance of absolute rest in bed for several days is clear' postinfarction..."[114]

Quite remarkably, Herrick managed to describe the world's first heart attack in 1912 and then, without missing a beat, he immediately knew that strict bed rest was an essential form of treatment – for a condition never before described. A clever trick don't you think? Also, a perfect example of the drive to do something, anything, rather than accept that he could not possibly know what the best course of action was.

In truth, strict bed rest for a few days may not have been too bad. Over time, however, Herricks' *several days* became a standard six weeks. Medical dogma then dictated that during this six week period if you allowed a patient to move a muscle this was virtual medical malpractice. To quote a prominent physician from the 1930s:

"The patient is to be guarded by day and night nursing and helped in every way to avoid voluntary movement, or effort."

Thomas Lewis

Now you can easily see the thinking here. After a heart attack the heart muscle is damaged, therefore it must be 'protected' from any extra strain. A five year old could tell you that. Yes, indeed, a five year old *could* tell you that.

Why six weeks? I suspect this time period slipped over from orthopaedics, where it generally takes a broken bone about six weeks to heal. Bones and heart muscle, pretty much the same thing aren't they? OK, no they're not, but let us not quibble. It's all different forms of bodily healing stuff isn't it? Sorry, you may have thought there was some science behind this.

Anyway, what started to emerge here was the perfect storm. The need to do something, anything, backed up by the simplest of simple hypotheses that anyone could understand. The heart must not be put under any strain after a heart attack. Why would anyone need to do a study on this? Bed rest is obviously beneficial, is it not?

To continue with Braunwald's sad little tale:

"...Unfortunately, 'a few days became six weeks,' Dr Braunwald observed, with a 30% in-patient mortality for acute myocardial infarction in his time of training. 'On early-morning rounds to draw bloods, I'd find that some of our patients had slipped away quietly in the night in some of the rooms off to the side,' he lamented."

A 30% in-patient mortality for acute myocardial infarction! I think that statement may need another two exclamation marks at least. The fact is that this death rate would have been slashed if those suffering a heart attack had stayed at home and started lifting concrete slabs from day one. I exaggerate, but not by very much. In fact, probably not at all.

The reality is that strict bed rest killed millions of people over a fifty year period from 1912 to around the mid 1960s. Then, all of a sudden the idea was shelved. Gone, as if it had never been.

If you think my estimate of 'millions' is an exaggeration, the truth is that I am probably being cautious. It was more like tens of millions. Just to start with one decade, in one country. In the 1950s in the USA around 2,000,000 men suffered a heart attack each and every year (this was the peak death rate in the US). About 40% died before they could reach hospital. The other 60% survived.

For the sake of simple maths I will round this 60% figure down to 50%. This leaves us with 1,000,000 men reaching hospital every year (I am removing women from this thought experiment). 300,000 of those men then died whilst in hospital.

Today about 8% of those reaching hospital will die. Medical interventions are estimated to have caused about half of the reduction from 30% to 8%. Which still leaves an unaccounted 11% being killed due to enforced bed rest. Or, 111,000 excess deaths per year, in the US alone. Or 1,100,000, in 1 decade.

Over a period of 50 years this is 5,500,000 premature deaths, in the US alone, and only for men. Worldwide, you could at least double, or treble this death toll. If you want to argue these figures, I am sure you could. However, you will still be left with millions and millions dead around the world... excluding women.

You may wonder how bed rest is so deadly. Well, there are two main ways it can kill you. First, lying in bed stationary for six weeks means that there is a damned good chance of developing a deep vein thrombosis (DVT) in the legs. A high percentage of these break off, travel to the lungs, and block the arteries in the lungs causing a pulmonary embolus (PE) – these carry a very high mortality rate.

Secondly, without any exercise, and especially after a heart attack, the heart degenerates very rapidly. It becomes weaker, and deadly heart rhythms develop, so you are far more likely to die of ventricular fibrillation, the condition we now zap with a defibrillator (which saves lives occasionally). Whatever the exact cause of death, hundreds of thousands were dying each year as a direct result of enforced bed rest.

All of that is terribly sad and, I believe, inarguable. However, with regard to this discussion, the most important part of this story is the fact that no-one noticed that anything untoward was happening. You may think that seems almost impossible. How can millions die without something appearing on the radar screen somewhere? I would turn the question round to ask. How *could* anyone notice?

People had heart attacks, then they went to hospital where they received the best possible care. Even with the best possible care, around 30% died. Without such care even more would die, wouldn't they? Imagine how bad it would have been if all these heart attack patients had got up and walked about after a couple of days. What idiot could suggest such a thing? Do you want them *all* to die!

In fact, as far as I am aware, no-one even began to question strict bed rest until, at least, the mid-1950s. If you look back through the historical literature on various medical practices you can normally find a few lonely voices raised against the prevailing dogma.

At the time these voices are, without exception, firmly squashed. But I find they almost always leave a few ghosts in the machine for those who have the patience to look back through the record. In this case there appears to have been almost total silence. It seems the idea of strict bed rest held everyone, and I mean everyone, in its thrall for at least 50 years.

Then, suddenly, strict bed rest was gone, never to be mentioned again. After killing far more people than died as a direct cause of warfare in the first and second world wars combined. Why did it disappear? Well that is a tale for another time. The Apollo moon mission played a major part, where young volunteers were asked to lie stationary in bed to mimic the lack of exercise in space. Six weeks later their hearts were working very poorly indeed.

At this point you might be thinking, why bother telling me about the terrible damage done by strict bed rest? Everyone who was going to die has died. Almost all the doctors who enforced bed rest are now dead, and this form of management is dead too. It can never do any more harm again.

All true, but the form of thinking that caused this terrible disaster still stalks the land. It is a combination of the emotional drive to *do* something or provide a solution combined with '*a very simple idea.*' This, I believe, is the catalyst for disaster. The next factor to add into this already toxic brew is the absolute certainty that what you are doing is right. A certainty which means that no-one even bothers to do a clinical trial before heading off at high speed to ensure that it becomes gold-standard treatment.

This pattern can be seen across a wide range of medical interventions that were once seen as an unquestionable good. For example, the radical mastectomy for breast cancer, or removal of toxic colon (for almost everything). Whenever, and wherever, you come across a combination of these three forces acting together I believe that you need to be on high alert.

Is there a new bed rest?

So where is the bed rest of today? Well, I believe that AIDS is one possible place to look. When AIDS first emerged, panic stalked the land, especially amongst the homosexual community. It appeared that thousands were suddenly dying from a terrible disease that had appeared from nowhere.

There was massive pressure to do something, anything. Remarkably quickly it was announced that AIDS was caused by the previously unknown Human Immunodeficiency Virus (HIV). It was immediately decreed that the way to treat AIDS was to obliterate this virus – or at least to prevent it from replicating itself within human cells.

This is tricky, as HIV is a retrovirus that is made by the DNA within the cell, and then appears to hide there. So you cannot get at it easily. In fact, most viruses are very difficult to attack with drugs, as they too hide. But HIV seems to hide better than most.

Wellcome, recognising that there was a potentially massive market, just begging for something to be done, dragged an anti-cancer drug from the shelf – one they just happened to have made earlier. This drug stopped cell (and viral) replication dead. It was called AZT. Research on AZT had actually been abandoned in the 1960s due to problems with terrible toxicity.

THE DEVELOPMENT OF AZT

In 1964, a chemist, Jerome Horwitz, synthesised a sophisticated experimental cell poison for the treatment of cancerous tumour cells. It was called Suramin, or Compound S. Its formal title is 3'-azido-3'-deoxythymidine zidovudine for short – but everyone knows it by its nickname, AZT.

It works like this. Thymidine is one of the four nucleotides (building blocks) of DNA, the basic molecule of life. AZT is an artificial fake, a dead ringer for thymidine. As a cell synthesises new DNA while preparing to divide in order to spawn another, AZT either steals in to take the place of the real thing, or else disrupts the delicate process by interfering with the cell's regulation of the relative concentrations of nucleotide pools present during DNA synthesis. That's the end of the cell line. Cell division and replication, wrecked by the presence of the plastic imposter, comes to a halt. Chemotherapeutic drugs

---

> *such as AZT are described as DNA chain terminators accordingly.*
> *Their effect is wholesale cell death of every type, particularly the rapidly di-*
> *viding cells of the immune system and those lining our guts. Horwitz found*
> *that the sick immune cells went, but with so many others that his poison was*
> *plainly useless as a medicine. It was akin to napalm-bombing a school to kill*
> *some roof-rats. AZT was abandoned. It wasn't even patented. For two dec-*
> *ades it collected dust, forgotten – until the advent of the AIDS era.*[115]

AZT was so horribly toxic that it wasn't even patented after being synthesised. Which should had given pause for thought. However, when faced with such a deadly epidemic, massive toxicity was better than inevitable and rapid death... was it not?

The thinking was simple. We have a virus replicating itself inside our bodies. Not only that, but it hides within white cells themselves – the very cells we use to fight infection. How to stop this cunning enemy? Simple, obliterate the process of DNA replication.

In theory this would stop HIV in its tracks. Very much the same thinking as used in the development of many anticancer agents. Cancer cells tend to divide more rapidly than any normal cell in the body. So, if you attack the process of replication you are likely to preferentially wipe out cancer cells. (Just be careful not to wipe out the rest of the body at the same time).

When it was studied, it was found that, unsurprisingly, AZT reduced the 'viral load' in AIDS. Frankly it would have been amazing if it had not, as all replication, of everything inside the human body, was being switched off.

Once this was demonstrated, Wellcome moved into top gear, and promoted the use of AZT with ruthless efficiency. No-one questioned whether or not this simple treatment might not be a good thing. As with many areas of medicine, an unstoppable momentum had built up, based on the need to do something, anything, combined with the simplest idea available.

AIDS is caused by HIV, HIV replicates inside humans cells, AZT stops DNA/viral replication, and AZT reduces the measurable viral load. Problem sorted. Not quite as simple as bed rest following an MI, but in reality the underlying concepts were not much more complex.

However, unlike the use of bed rest in acute MI, some attempts were made to see if AZT actually worked. Unfortunately, there was mass hysteria surrounding AIDS at the time of the first trial. The homosexual lobby protested long and loud that it was unethical to withhold treatment that might work from anyone. This meant that the first placebo controlled trial was, effectively, sabotaged.

It is true that the data from this first study did look very promising. 19 died in the placebo arm, and only 1 in the AZT arm. As the investigators reported:

"These data demonstrate that AZT administration can decrease mortality and the frequency of opportunistic infections in a selected group of subjects with AIDS or AIDS–related complex, at least over the 8 to 24 weeks of observation in this study."[116]

However, as the researchers went on to say:

"When the study was terminated, 27 subjects had completed 24 weeks of the study, 152 had completed 16 weeks, and the remainder had completed at least 8 weeks."

The reality is that only 15 patients (5% of the total) had completed even 24 weeks of treatment. 23 patients were treated for less than 4 weeks. On average, patients had received treatment for about 17 weeks at the time the study was aborted. In short, the study was horribly incomplete and terminated early – which is always a terribly bad idea.

Also, during this very short time period, 8% of participants died in 17 weeks. This was a catastrophically high mortality rate, and cannot possibly represent what is going to happen to the average person contracting AIDS. At least one would certainly hope not.

These issues, which would be enough to condemn most studies to the dustbin, were only the tip of the iceberg. Many of those taking part in the study took their tablets to friendly chemists in order to analyse them and find out if they were on the active substance or not. Some of those, knowing they were taking a placebo, started to import AZT from Mexico to take themselves. (Which could, I suppose, account for the 8% mortality rate).

In addition, many of those on the study started communicating amongst themselves to find out who was taking the drug, or the placebo, and then began swapping tablets between each other. The 'blinding' of the study also fell apart on the researcher's side. Through the effects of AZT on red blood cells, it was easy to spot who was taking the medication, and who was not.

Which means that, for reasons not within the control of the investigators, this attempt to run a double-blind placebo-controlled study, turned into an unscientific mess. Recognising the catastrophic flaws of this study another major trial was done, right? Wrong. When it comes to the treatment of AIDS this was both the first, and the only, placebo-controlled study. Yup, ladies and gentlemen, that's it.

And upon this single study rests all other AIDS drug treatments since developed. You may wonder how this can possibly be. Well, the benefits of antiretroviral medication are now established beyond doubt. So much so that it would be considered unethical to carry out a placebo controlled study. Yes, I know, this does not make any sense.

Actually, it does make sense if you are willing to believe that the initial AZT study proved beyond a shadow of doubt that antiretroviral medication works. I would put it to you that if I ran a study containing fewer than 300 people, in which only 5% completed the full trial protocol, whilst participants in the placebo and treatment arms merrily swapped drugs between themselves and imported drugs from Mexico, I believe I would struggle to get it published. In fact, I know I would *not* get it published. (For a far more detailed analysis of the many flaws of this study see this reference.[117])

What I do know is the following. If AZT caused more damage and deaths than placebo, then we are now in the six weeks of bed rest scenario again. Everyone gets drug treatment for AIDS, no-one does not (apart from the easily dismissed nutcases who think it may not be that good).

Yes, we know that the newer drug regimens such as highly active antiretroviral therapy (HAART) are much better than AZT. That much, at least, seems certain. But so what? It may be that HAART is simply the equivalent of three weeks bed rest, rather than six. Deadly, but not as deadly.

The next result of all of this is that, as with bed rest, we now just 'know' that various antiretroviral drugs are keeping people alive. To suggest otherwise is to suffer the Duesberg fate. Or the fate of Matthias Rath. To be dismissed as dangerous, Nazi-sympathizing, racist, mass murderers. I suspect this may also become the Kendrick fate after this book is published. But hey, that's the way it is. Water, let me introduce you to a duck's back.

Having just said this, I should mention that another AZT study called Concorde was done a few years later. This did not compare AZT with a placebo, but it was a close as anything else has got. It compared the effect of starting AZT early, rather than waiting to start it later. It was also done in people who had no actual symptoms of AIDS, just disease markers, so they were a much 'healthier' population than the 1987 study.

It was reported by the coordinating committee in *The Lancet* in April 1994 (for placebo read 'started AZT later'):

"A total of 172... participants died [169 while taking AZT, 3 while on placebo]... The results of Concorde do not encourage the early use of zidovudine in symptom-free HIV-infected adults."[118]

I have to admit that this trial was far from perfect, as it was not a placebo-controlled study. It was a study of early vs. late treatment. But it does strongly suggest that the sooner you took AZT, the more likely you were to die early, despite the fact that the disease 'markers' were greatly improved.

All of which means that, when you get down to basics, we have one horribly flawed study suggesting AZT may be much better than placebo. We have another, far larger and better controlled study, suggesting early AZT treatment may be much worse than late AZT treatment. Which may be another way of demonstrating that AZT is far more harmful than placebo. Where does this leave us? In a very difficult place. If AZT was, and remains, worse for AIDS sufferers than doing nothing, how could we now establish this? Well we can't.

Equally, how can we know that the newer drugs, and drugs regimes, actually work? Well, we can't, because no-one will ever do a placebo controlled study ever again. We only know that the newer drugs are far better than AZT, which, of course, might have been killing people.

Anyway, returning to the main theme here. With AIDS I believe that the main problem was that we had the deadly trinity in play once again:

- The need to do something/anything;

- Grabbing the simple/easy hypothesis too early;

- Being so certain your hypothesis is correct you don't do any study to prove that it is beneficial – you just get on with it.

So, yes, I do believe that patterns of poor behaviour/thinking can be seen today. Of course, when you see these patterns it does not always mean that something is a terrible idea. No-one did clinical trials on hip replacements – which are a fantastic operation. No-one did clinical trials on penicillin – you didn't really need to, dying soldiers were given penicillin and stopped dying. No-one has done a controlled clinical study on the damage that smoking does – but you don't really need to. No one has done a clinical study on pushing people out of planes without parachutes to see if they may save lives... ditto.

However, if you start doing things that are not based on controlled studies you must always be alert to the possibility that what you are doing may actually be harmful. The medical profession, sadly, becomes exceedingly defensive if someone dares to question the benefit of established forms of treatment. The powers that be ignore, dismiss, attack, and the attacks can become highly personal. Usually you are accused of killing people. (I have no doubt whatsoever that my example of AIDS treatment will result in such attacks when all I am suggesting is that you go and check out the original data and decide for yourself).

If you want to really depress yourself, read up on the history of the radical mastectomy for the treatment of breast cancer. This procedure was introduced by Halsted in the late nineteenth century. It rapidly became *the* treatment of choice. It was never trialled, it was never reviewed. It was just considered to be the best, indeed, the only thing to do.

How could you argue against removing the tumour, the breast, the other breast, most lymph glands and half the chest wall. Sadly, almost anything that could be removed, was removed. Of course it was horribly disfiguring and painful. But you could not risk leaving even the smallest part of a tumour behind – could you. As it turns out, yes you could – indeed should.

I remember when I was a medical student, being part of a ward round taken by the Professor of Surgery in Aberdeen. He proudly introduced us to a woman on whom he had just operated, carrying out a radical mastectomy. Afterwards I mentioned to him that I had read that less radical forms of surgery may be just as effective as the radical mastectomy.

Let me just say that my observation was not met with instant acceptance. A wide ranging discussion on the latest research did not ensue. Afterwards a fellow student opined that I had been very brave to bring up the issue, and then asked if I was alright. I replied that I had certainly had better days, having just been subjected to a ten minute attack of pure poisonous bile – during which it was made very clear what said professor intended to do to my career in medicine.

I think my fellow students who witnessed that attack all made a quiet mental note to themselves. 'Do *not* question current medical treatment. Repeat. Do *not* question current medical treatment.' It is generally not a great career move. Unless you fancy a career selling the *Big Issue*, that is.

I suppose the anger of the professor was perfectly understandable. Doctors want to believe they are doing things that are of real benefit to patients. Otherwise how could they continue to act? If someone comes breezing along and tells them that, not only are you doing no good, you are actually killing people or disfiguring them unnecessarily. Well, they are not likely to open their arms wide and accept that their professional life has been a complete, damaging, waste of time.

Our sense of our own value is jealously guarded. We will play endless games to avoid facing up to reality – if that reality is too painful to bear. Unfortunately this makes medicine less open to new ideas than most other areas. You can be wrong about the existence, or otherwise, of dark matter and no-one is going to live or die. Get it wrong about the treatment of heart attacks and millions can and indeed did die.

Anyway, without plunging too deeply in the darkness that is human psychology, it is time to move back to the main theme here. Trying to spot current medical activities that may be doing more harm than good.

Coronary artery bypass grafting

In truth, I believe it would be possible to write several books on current examples of medical treatments, and ideas, that are very widespread, that could be doing harm. However, I will restrict myself to three more potential examples:

- Coronary artery bypass grafting;

- Polypharmacy QoF;

- Bariatric surgery.

First to look at Coronary Artery Bypass Graft (CABG), often pronounced 'cabbage.'

As we know, the event that kills most people with a heart attack (myocardial infarction), is a blockage of one or more of the coronary arteries, which are the arteries that supply the heart with blood. This interrupts the oxygen supply to a large section of heart muscle, and the affected muscle is liable to die – or 'infarct'. (Actually the heart muscle does not die, it converts to a form of scar tissue, but that is an issue for another day).

Clearly, it would be best to try to stop this happening in the first place. But how *can* you stop this happening in the first place? Well it was decided that the best way to do this, is to identify whether or not a coronary artery is dangerously narrowed. If so, you then 'bypass' that artery with another healthy and fully patent (unobstructed) blood vessel from somewhere else in the body. At first this was usually a vein from the leg.

Once you have added a bypass, the blood can flow freely past any future obstruction and this will 'obviously' save your life. You can have single, double, triple and quadruple bypasses, depending on how many blocked arteries you are trying to bypass.

The way to identify which arteries are dangerously narrowed is to stick a probe/catheter into an artery in the groin, push it up to the heart, and then direct it into the coronary arteries themselves. At which point you inject a bit of dye and do a low intensity x-ray to visualise the artery concerned. This is known as angiography, and it shows up narrowings and obstructions pretty clearly.

Of course, if you do have an angiogram, which shows a 70% blockage, what would you do? You'd say, bypass that sucker, straight away. (In fact some cardiologists actually refer to an obstruction of the Left Anterior Descending (LAD) artery as *The widowmaker.* Hmmm, no pressure there then.) Otherwise you are living with an unexploded bomb in your chest – are you not? The correct answer is... maybe, maybe not.

As you may have guessed, the CABG was instantly adopted worldwide as *the* major life saving operation for people with 'dangerously' narrowed coronary arteries. Cardiovascular surgeons became blindingly rich doing them, patients were as grateful as grateful could be, and remained so for years. 'You saved my life doc.' etc.

Once again, we can see the dreaded trinity in action:

- The need to do something/anything;

- Grabbing the simple/easy hypothesis too early;

- Being so certain your hypothesis is correct you don't do any study to prove that it is beneficial – you just get on with it.

"For every complex problem there is an answer that is clear, simple, and wrong."
H. L. Mencken

You think there were controlled clinical trials on CABG? Well, think again. There were none. Zip, nada. Who would bother to study something so obvious, so simple, and so brilliant and, to top it all off, just so fabulously lucrative. Come on, get with the programme man.

One man who did not get with the programme was Bernard Lown, a cardiologist who should be famous around the world... but is significantly less famous than he should be.

Bernard Lown, M.D. was born in 1921 in Lithuania. He was the original developer of the defibrillator and a founder of the International Physicians for the Prevention of Nuclear War. This organisation was awarded the Nobel Peace Prize in 1985 for its work against nuclear pro-liferation. Lown Cardiovascular Center in Brookline, MA, is named after him and Lown also has a bridge named in his honor in the twin cities of Lewiston and Auburn, Maine.

Lown is still alive – at the time of writing. Here is a small section from a blog he has written on the matter of CABG, and angiography, and the whole mess that this area became:

"Forty years ago I stopped referring most patients with stable coronary heart disease (CHD) for cardiac angiography. This procedure permits visualizing the extent of obstructed coronary arteries. What occasioned my deviation? The problem was that nearly all those undergoing angiography ended up having surgery, namely, coronary artery bypass grafting, or CABG (pronounced "cabbage").

"What could be wrong with improving blood flow to the heart by unblocking an obstructed or narrowed artery? Such a seemingly common sense approach would have had the approval of every plumber who encounters a blocked faucet."

Indeed, this process would have had the approval of every plumber, every five year old child and thus, virtually all cardiologists. However, blood vessels are not merely pipes, the heart is not simply a pump, and the body is not an inanimate object. Treating atherosclerosis simply as a disorder of the plumbing system is certainly simple and straightfor-ward, and easy to understand. It is also utterly stupid.

A relative of mine has no patent (unobstructed) coronary arteries. None. Yet, though he is now very elderly, he walks around without trou-ble, goes upstairs without any great difficulty, and has no angina. Yes, I shall repeat that, he has no patent coronary arteries, and he is still alive and well, and walking about. This is possible because his heart grew additional blood vessels to get round the blockages caused by smoking.

The development of these new blood vessels is called collateral circu-lation. You may be surprised to know that the process of developing new blood vessels to get round obstructions is not in the least unusual. It is present in many millions of human hearts around the world. It is some-thing that living organisms, such as humans, can do to protect themselves from harm caused by narrow blood vessels. It is nature's very own CABG.

However, such knowledge had precisely no impact on the charge of the cardiology brigade charge towards the world of the CABG. I don't know if cardiologists are particularly prone to simplistic thinking, but it sometimes seems so.

'This man has had a heart attack... ' 'OMG, he must rest for six weeks to protect the heart.'

'This man has narrowed arteries in the heart... ' 'OMG, we must bypass them with other blood vessels.'

'This man has narrowed arteries in the heart...' 'OMG, we must open up the narrowings... '

Yes, after the CABG came the balloon and the stent. A balloon is a device whereby you insert a catheter into the coronary artery. Once you reach the narrow bit you blow up the balloon at the end and drag it backwards, forcing the artery to open up. Yes, I know. Ouch. (Actually, it is pain free).

This was about as effective as you might imagine as the arteries rapidly closed up again. So, very clever people then developed an open latticed metal pipe called a stent. This was stuck on the end of a catheter, taken to the point of narrowing then released. At which point the narrowed artery was forced open, and the internal metal 'stent' kept it open.

In many places this has now taken over from the CABG as the 'operation de jour.' It was, of course, thoroughly tested in many clinical studies before it was introduced. Ho... ho. Not.

That, however, is running ahead of myself. Getting back to CABG. We have an operation done on millions of people, where at no point did anyone, ever, check whether the outcomes were better than not operating. No studies done... ever.

Bernard Lown felt that this was not a good idea. He had seen previously healthy people have major strokes following angiography. He also knew that the operative mortality was in the order of 2-5%. It was also clear that many bypasses blocked up quite quickly after the operation. In short, a lot of harm was caused, and many bypasses didn't last long before they, too, completely furred up again.

To quote Lown once more:

"In the 1970s coronary bypass grafting was the only available approach for directly dealing with an obstructed vessel. CABG, as already stated, was not innocuous. It carried a 2 to 5 percent operative mortality. The grafts tended to clot and obstruct. Ten years after the operation a majority had reoccluded. Reoperation was then associated with double-digit mortality.

"Nearly 10 percent of patients undergoing CABG experienced some complications. Blood clots dislodged during the operation resulted in strokes and heart attacks. Undetected by cardiologists for many years was the impaired intellectual function afflicting many. It manifested in subtle memory losses and mild depression.

"I missed these complications until alerted by several spouses of patients. As one succinctly stated, 'My husband is physically normal, but he isn't the guy I married.' Surprisingly it took a decade or longer for these disabilities to be recognized. A published study on magnetic resonance imaging found that 51 per cent of those who had CABG demonstrated some brain damage."[119]

Could the benefits, if there were any, be so great as to trump the significant harm done? Bernard Lown tried to do studies in this area to find out, but immediately faced enormous difficulties. The main problem was simple, but very difficult to surmount. The moment someone had angiography which highlighted a narrowed artery, they wanted an operation, straight away. No *widowmaker* for me, thanks very much.

The idea that you could enter people into a study after angiography and ask them not to have CABG just did not work. No-one would agree to go into the 'non CABG' arm of the study. This is similar to the situation with AIDS, where AZT became the standard life-saving treatment so quickly that not prescribing AZT was tantamount to medical malpractice. Even though there was no real evidence that it actually worked.

Enter a Kafkasque world which goes something like this.

You don't know for sure if someone has occluded coronary arteries until you do an angiogram. Once you have demonstrated that the arteries are occluded, the patient is so terrified they are going to die that they demand a CABG. This means that you cannot run a study with a 'standard treatment' arm. This means that a controlled study is impossible. Perfect. Get out of that.

What Bernard Lown tried to do was to establish ways of diagnosing coronary artery obstruction clinically, without doing an angiogram. You could then put people into two groups, CABG, or standard medical treatment:

"We therefore determined to study stable CHD patients having advanced disease without subjecting them to angiographic investigation. Without viewing the coronary anatomy, how could we be certain that the selected patients had advanced disease? An extensive cardiovascular literature affirmed that the capacity to exercise on a motorized treadmill and the ensuing electrocardiographic changes indicated the severity of coronary vessel obstructions...

"In the first of four studies we carried out over the ensuing thirty years, we recruited 144 consecutive patients with advanced coronary artery disease. These were followed for an average period of nearly five years, during which time 11

patients died, for an annual rate of 1.4 percent. We referred only 9 patients for CABG (1.3 percent annually). These results were better than the best outcomes being reported for those undergoing CABG. We concluded that resorting to cardiac surgery was infrequently indicated for patients with stable CHD."

What happened at this point? Well, have a wild guess. They struggled for four years to get their results published. Why, because they didn't do angiography. Not doing angiography meant that the study was considered critically flawed.

"It took four years before the New England Journal of Medicine published our findings. A flurry of angry letters followed with the recurrent motif that without coronary angiography our conclusions were invalid."

I love the irony here. CABG was introduced on the back of absolutely no evidence whatsoever. When someone tries to provide some evidence, they are castigated because their study did not do angiography, which meant that their evidence was of poor quality. Unlike the very high quality evidence that was used to start the whole CABG bandwagon rolling... not!

I am afraid that a great deal of medicine is much like this. A form of management is introduced because it is simple, and seems like a damned good idea. It then becomes the 'gold standard' for treatment of that condition. At which point it becomes impossible, or unethical, to do a study to prove whether or not it actually works.

Of course CABGs are still being done. Why? Well, there was on old first world war song that the troops used to sing to the tune of Old Lang Syne. It explained what they were doing in France, being machine gunned to death by the Germans. *'We're here because we're here because we're here because we're here. We're here because we're here because we're here because we're here... rpt.'* to change the words slightly. *'We CABG because we CABG because we CABG because we CABG... rpt.'*

Leaving CABG behind. What is the latest form of 'treatment' to be introduced on the back of the deadly trinity?

Polypharmacy

It is not a current treatment, it is polypharmacy. By which I mean the prescribing of many different drugs, all at the same time, mainly to the elderly. It is a particularly acute problem in the UK where the Department of Health introduced a complex system of targets that doctors strive to attain. It goes under the banner of the Quality Outcome Framework (QoF).

I am not going into the Byzantine structure of QoF in any great detail – as it is incredibly complex and depressing. However, reducing it to basics, it has been decreed that doctors should measure a whole series of 'risk factors' for various diseases e.g. blood pressure, cholesterol, blood sugar levels, obesity, etc. etc. If the measures are high, bring them down (see Chapter Five).

In addition, if someone has had a heart attack, or stroke, or thought to have had, guidelines state that they need to be put on a whole series of different drugs as preventative treatment. This usually includes three different antihypertensives, a blood thinner, and a statin. This happens even if a heart attack has not actually been diagnosed.

In one of the units I work, where elderly patients undergo rehabilitation, the average number of medications that the patients are taking is 10.2. This is up from 9.6 last year. Apart from the ubiquitous blood-pressure lowering meds, over 90% take a statin, almost all are on drugs for osteoporosis (thin bones), most take an antiacid drug and at least 50% are on diabetic medication – usually two or three different drugs.

In order to save me time writing out the drug charts I am working on a great big stamp that has all the regular drugs engraved on it. Simvastatin 40mg 1 tab (nocte), clopidogrel 75mg 1 tab mane, bendroflumethaizide 5mg 1 tab mane, Alendronic acid 70mg I tab weekly etc. etc etcetera, etcetera rpt. Bam! 'All standard drug therapy prescribed, sir!'

Now you can make a case – although not a terribly powerful one – that each of these medications has some benefit. An ACE inhibitor after a heart attack has some barely significant benefits, as does a beta-blocker. However, you cannot provide any data to show that a beta-blocker, a statin, an anticoagulant and metformin and a sulphonylurea have any benefits when given together. No evidence at all.

Why not? You've guessed it, because a study has not been done, in truth *never* will be done, on the effects of giving four or five different drugs together. It is assumed that if drug x provides 1% benefit and drug y provides 1% benefit and drug z provides 1% benefit that, if you add them together, you will get:

X (1% benefit) + Y (1% benefit) + Z (1% benefit) = 3% (benefit)

Simple idea? Yes, it could not be any simpler – could it? No, it could not. My pet goldfish understood it without the slightest difficulty. At least I think it did. Maybe that little O it made with its mouth wasn't actually agreement. Just stunned surprise that humans could be more stupid than he, my pet goldfish, a.k.a.... Albert Einstein.

Sorry. I think I may be getting a little too facetious. But when faced with thinking like this I often find myself resorting to mockery.

Could it possibly be, just possibly, that if you stick 10 different drugs into an elderly person that the adverse effects, and inevitable drug interactions, may possibly, just possibly, overwhelm any possible benefits? If so, should you not then have attempted to do a study on this issue before imposing polypharmacy on every single living person in the population?

The Quality Outcome Framework in the UK is by far the greatest experiment on human health ever attempted. The only problem with it is that we will never, ever, be able to know if it works or not. Are people being made more healthy, or are they being killed? Is QoF the equivalent of six weeks of bed rest?

We purport to be in a Brave New World of evidence based healthcare, whereby we only do things that are supported by high quality evidence... hollow laughter. Yet, the UK has introduced the most massive healthcare intervention ever without a molecule of evidence to support it. It is also costing billions – that could be spent on stuff that we know actually works.

You may wonder if there is any evidence that polypharmacy might be damaging. Yes, of course there is. There is even a paper called "The war against polypharmacy: a new cost-effective geriatric-palliative approach for improving drug therapy in disabled elderly people". This documented a 2007 study from Israel comparing 119 disabled patients in 6 geriatric nursing departments with a control group of 71 patients of comparable age, gender and co-morbidities in the same wards.[120] A total of 332 different drugs were discontinued in 119 patients (an average of 2.8 drugs per patient). This was not associated with significant adverse effects. After one year, the mortality rate was 45% in the control group but only 21% in the study group. The patients' annual referral rate to acute care facilities was 30% in the control group but only 11.8% in the study group. The intervention was associated with a substantial decrease in the cost of drugs.

The researchers concluded: "*Application of the geriatric-palliative methodology in the disabled elderly enables simultaneous discontinuation of several medications and yields a number of benefits: reduction in mortality rates and referrals to acute care facilities, lower costs, and improved quality of living.*"

The first thing to say here is that, if there ever was a 'war' against polypharmacy, then polypharmacy won a long time ago... at least in the UK.

For those who find scientific papers somewhat opaque, the key point from this paper is the following:

The one year mortality in those who did *not* have their medications reduced was **45%**;

The one year mortality in those who did have their medications reduced was **21%**.

This has more than halved overall mortality in a single year. Which is a better result than I have seen for any drug intervention, ever, anywhere. So it would seem that the best possible drug treatment discovered... is to stop taking drugs. As an added bonus you save lots of money, and make the patient feel much better, all at the same time.

Just one paper? No, of course not. There are a number of different studies demonstrating that discontinuing medication particularly in the elderly is a good thing to do. A review paper in the *Journal of the American Medical Association* (*JAMA*) came to the following conclusions:

"The finding that simultaneous discontinuation of many drugs is not associated with significant risks and apparently improves quality of life should encourage physicians to consider testing this in larger RCTs (randomised controlled studies) across a variety of medical cultural settings. Polypharmacy may have different faces in different countries or clinics but there is no doubt that the problem is global. This approach has international relevance; it combines our best existing evidence with patient-focused care while actively avoiding extrapolation from inappropriate populations where no evidence exists for treatment in elderly patients."[121]

In fact, I cannot find any evidence that polypharmacy, however you define it, does anything but harm. In the face of such evidence what did the UK authorities decide to do? Why, they set about to create a system designed to drive the biggest explosion of polypharmacy ever seen. What else would you expect them to do? They are, after all, experts – are they not?

Of course some drugs cannot be stopped, as they are vital. Insulin in patients with type I diabetes for example. But the vast majority of medications that the elderly are taking can clearly cause harm. Blood pressure medications often cause very low blood pressure on standing up (postural hypotension), and this can greatly increase falls risk. Elderly people falling are likely to break hips, and broken hips are not good things.

In fact, in one of my current jobs, I spend a lot of time taking people off as many meds as I can. In many cases this has resulted in spectacular improvements in overall health and well-being. Of course I know that as soon as they are discharged, and head back to their own GP, all drugs will be restarted in order to meet QoF targets. Blah!

Another issue here that I think is extremely important is that all this endless prescribing of more and more drugs has been done on the basis of clinical studies on much younger people with only one illness (no co-morbidities). So slamming them into an elderly population with three or four different medical conditions is a complete leap into the unknown.

To quote the *JAMA* paper again:

"Drugs are often given to older people based on studies of younger persons without significant comorbidity who have a life expectancy of several decades. Applying the results and/or the clinical guidelines developed from these studies to elderly patients is inappropriate because of higher risk to benefit ratios with increased age, comorbidity, disability, and number of medications prescribed."

Inappropriate... Quite. A good word, but I can think of several better ones.

So why are bigger and more definitive studies not done in this area? Well, it will not surprise you to know that pharmaceutical companies are not exactly straining at the leash to fund clinical studies showing that the more drugs that you take, the shorter and more miserable your life will be. Without industry funding such a study would be financially beyond most researchers.

Also, most researchers know full well upon which side of the bread the butter is spread. If you discover that prescribing more and more drugs causes harm, you will find yourself on the side of the bread that is entirely a 'butter free' zone. A zone where invites to international conferences, whilst staying at five – sorry four star hotels now the new guidance has come in, can only be glimpsed through the Hubble space telescope – at a range of 12,000 light years. It's life Jim, but not as we know it.

Just in case you think I am a lonely madman, tilting against wind-mills, here is what Dr Des Spence has to say about QoF. He is a GP in Scotland and writes for the *British Medical Journal* – from whence this paragraph has been lifted:

"The QoF simply hasn't worked. It is a bureaucratic disaster, measuring the measurable but eroding the all-important immeasurable, and squandering our time, effort and money. It has made patients of us all and turned skilled clini-

cians into bean counters. Incentives and centralised targets are under scrutiny throughout the public sectors because targets just lead to gaming. It's time to look away from the screen and at the patient once again. Turn off the financial life support and let this failed initiative die."[122]

He goes on to point out that QoF has created 3,000,000 new statin users, over 10 years with no discernible effect on heart disease trends. Also, there has been no change in the trajectory of UK life expectancy. So, a great success then.

The response from the department of health is exactly what you would expect. Tighten the targets, introduce a whole series of new drug targets, and make everyone work harder and harder to achieve a world of blanket polypharamcy.

Question: Does the QoF = six weeks of bed rest?

Answer:We will never know, because no-one will ever do a controlled study on it

However, sometimes we can glimpse a flash of lightning in the black void. Here is an article from the *Daily Mail* in 2013

"Health officials are investigating a sudden rise in death rates in the elderly, particularly among women. Around 600 more people – mainly elderly – have died every week so far this year compared with the average for the last five years, official figures show.

"Since early 2012 there have been 23,400 more deaths than would have been expected in England and Wales. Officials from Public Health England – the new body responsible for monitoring disease – is investigating whether it is due to a particularly aggressive form of new viruses.

"But other experts believe it may be down to cuts to council care budgets, longer waits in A&E or even the elderly feeling they are a 'burden' to society during times of austerity. A report by Public Health England – obtained by Health Service Journal – states that 2013 is on course to be 'noticeably worse than any recent year".[123]

As you can guess, no mention is made anywhere that this could be due to the very drugs prescribed to keep them alive. The ever more aggressive drug therapy being shovelled down old people's throats. However, I know what I think. Watch this space whilst people dance around in an ever greater frenzy, avoiding the issue of polypharmacy's more spectacularly complex ways.

Bariatric surgery

As with almost all surgical interventions, bariatric surgery was started without a single controlled randomised study being done. It was carried out, it helped people to lose weight, it was good.

Before getting into this area in more detail, I should make it clear that surgery stands in its own unique place in medical interventions. A surgeon thinks a procedure is a good idea. They do it. End of.

In fairness, one of the reasons why this is not completely unreasonable is that is very difficult to do a randomised study on something that has never been done before. When you are doing the first procedure on humans, e.g. a heart transplant, very little testing is possible. You can practise your surgical technique on animals, but it isn't really the same thing.

Which means that with completely new operations, you are most definitely entering an unknown world. As most people know, the first heart transplant patient died shortly after the operation, as did the next few. The first kidney transplant patient did not live long. A number of life-saving surgical interventions started off by killing everyone they were tried on. Surgeons, and their support teams, often have to get good at performing new operations before any benefit ensues.

If you had done a randomised controlled clinical study on aortic valve replacement after the first ten attempts, then it would never have been allowed, ever again. Today this is a life-extending, and life-enhancing, procedure.

Unlike drug treatments, surgical operations can start very badly and then the outcomes gradually improve. Not just due to better technique, but there will also be improvements in anaesthetics, life support, heart lung machines, post-operative medications etc.

In short, surgery is a very different beast to a drug treatment. It is a constantly moving target. It is generally an improving target, but not always. For example, it did not matter how technically proficient a surgeon became at doing a radical mastectomy it remains disfiguring, damaging and pointless. The commonest operation in the 1920s was removal of the 'toxic' colon. This was an utterly useless operation that achieved nothing – except harm – however technically perfect the operation itself became.

If we want to look at surgery objectively, therefore, we need to look at the overall purpose of the surgery, rather than the technical skills of the surgical team. A 'good' operation done badly needs to be made better. A 'bad' operation, done well, is still a bad operation.

Which takes me back to bariatric surgery. Where, again the deadly trinity is in play.

- The need to do something/anything;

- Grabbing the simple/easy hypothesis too early;

- Being so certain your hypothesis is correct you don't do any study to prove that it is beneficial – you just get on with it.

There is no doubt that obesity is an increasing health problem. No drug or dietary interventions have achieved anything worth talking about. Yes, despite all the endless messages about 'healthy eating', and the vast explosion in nutritionists, dieticians, diet books, and new diets, people are getting fatter. (Cause, or association... I go for cause).

Something, therefore, 'had to be done'. Enter the surgeons to the sound of trumpets. *'The best way to get people to lose weight is to obliterate their stomachs,'* cried the surgeons. This, after wiring jaws together turned out to be a spectacular failure. *'Without a stomach, you must lose weight.'*

Of course, a stomachectomy (complete removal of the stomach) would be a bit on the drastic side. Evolution didn't just create the stomach for a laugh you know. It does have a function, indeed several functions. Also, attempting to attach the oesophagus directly to the duodenum would not work very well. A bit too much tension I would imagine. A bit like that point at the petrol station when you realise that the pump nozzle will not reach your petrol tank however hard you pull it.

Which means that various techniques have been developed to make the stomach smaller, in various ways. In some cases a big band is placed round the stomach, squeezing it, and turning it into a much smaller stomach. A gastric band.

Increasingly common is the 'gastric bypass'. This term describes series of different operations that reduce the volume of the stomach so you cannot eat a great deal before feeling full – and stopping. (The stomach is not entirely bypassed).

Although technically challenging, the underlying idea behind bariatric surgery couldn't be any simpler. However, unlike many of the interventions I have described up to now it most certainly works, at least it works on one level. People do lose weight, often dramatically. I suppose it would be kind of stunning if they did not. Also, there is nothing else on offer that is remotely effective in helping people to lose weight. So, where's the problem, exactly?

Well, if you are doing the operation purely for cosmetic reasons i.e. to make people look thinner and more attractive... then bariatric surgery must be counted as an unmitigated success. But if you doing it for health reasons then, hold on. Remember this wee graph?

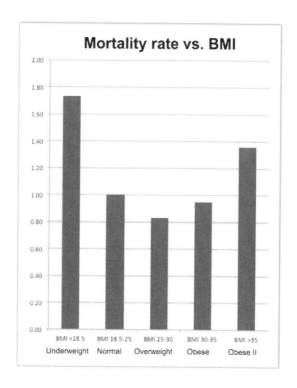

Everyone believes that obesity is incredibly damaging to health and at the extreme end, it is. However, the reality is that obesity is less of a health hazard than most people believe. Indeed, as you can see, the most dangerous body mass index is below 18.5. A level which would include all supermodels, and many 'athletes.' So, how about weight gain surgery instead? You know it makes sense.

No chance. Obesity is the great health scare of our age (picture a scene of people running about wildly, waving their hands in terror) and the tidal wave of weight loss operations continues unabated. At the time of writing there were, in the previous year, 200,000 bariatric operations done in the USA alone. Now that is a hell of a lot of operations. At around $30,000 a pop, we are talking six billion dollars a year – minimum.

Of course, money is not everything. What of the health benefits?

Well, perhaps I will start with the downsides. All major operations come with a mortality rate. In short, some people will certainly die as a direct result of being operated on. How many? Well difficult to tell. Data on operative mortality and morbidity are notoriously flexible.

Some time ago I was looking at the rates of post-operative wound infections across Europe. These rates varied from 0% to 20%. On the face of it, some surgeons appeared brilliant, others far less so. However, when you looked into the data in more detail, what seemed black and white merged into grey.

There were far too many issues to bore you with here, but just to give you a flavour of some of the difficulties. First, many surgeons would not classify anything as a post-operative infection if the patient had been discharged from their ward. So if a patient had an operation, and was moved elsewhere in the hospital, then an infection occurred, this was not recorded as having anything to do with 'their' operation. It was classified as a new, coincidental, infection.

Secondly, some hospitals required that a wound had to actually break down, and split open, before it was recorded as a post-operative infection. Others would record any redness and swelling as a post-operative infection. And so it went on.

As a piece of research it was fascinating, but utterly useless for proving anything. It was very clear that some surgeons will play the most fantastical games to prove that their operations were a most splendid success, with no complications of any sort. Death at home, a month after an operation, would not enter the statistics at all. That would be considered an unrelated 'community' death – even if they bled to death from the wound site.

Ah, hospital statistics on morbidity and mortality. A world of confused, mislabelled, game playing, nonsense.

My experience of digging into the data on surgical complications means that I am very wary of taking surgical morbidity and mortality figures at face value. However, some years ago I was pointed towards a review of bariatric surgery, and mortality in the *Journal of the American Medical Association*. A paper published in 2005. This looked at mortality rates from 16,000 patients undergoing bariatric surgery, with an average age under 50. The conclusions were:

The actual figures for all patients were that, one year after surgery, 4.6% of patients were dead. If you were a man, things were far worse. Within one year of surgery 7.5% were dead. Or to put this anther way. 1 out of 14 men undergoing weight loss surgery had died 1 year later. That is a pretty spectacular mortality rate.

I know that I will be told that this was just one study, and that this mortality rate was exceptionally high, '*we are now much better at doing this surgery, lessons have been learnt*' etc. All the usual guff. Maybe this is true, maybe not, after all this study did look at 16,000 patients. In truth, there have been very few controlled studies done in this area. The vast majority of studies have compared one form of surgery against another, to see which is better.

Of course, it is not just dying that is a problem with bariatric surgery. Wrapping a tight constricting band round someone's stomach, or bypassing the stomach in convoluted ways creates a wide range of problems, from malnutrition to destruction of the small bowel.

A small bowel transplant. Not exactly what you want to happen. I have also seen many reports of Korsakoff's dementia with significant neuropathy following bariatric surgery. Which is not exactly surprising as, without, a stomach you will not absorb critical vitamins and minerals, such as vitamin B1.

What is Korsakoff's dementia? I hear you ask. It's a neurological disorder named after Sergei Korsakoff, a Russian neuropsychiatrist, who described it during the late 19th century. Korsakoff's dementia is also called Korsakoff's syndrome, Korsakoff's psychosis, or amnesic-confabulatory syndrome and it is caused by a lack of thiamine (vitamin B1) in the brain. Its onset is linked to chronic alcohol abuse and/or severe malnutrition. If you have read about the increased incidence of alcohol abuse following bariatric surgery you may now be hearing a penny drop.

Korsakoff's syndrome is seen with *severe malnutrition.* We chop people's stomachs apart, and they become – effectively – malnourished. It may also interest you to know that Alzheimer's disease is closely associated with a lack of B vitamins.

A recent study showed that impaired supply of Vitamin B reduces cerebral atrophy. For the first time, a method has been found to protect those areas of the brain that are damaged by Alzheimer's disease.[126]

Just imagine if bariatric surgery, by significantly impairing the absorption of various B vitamins, were to increase the risk of developing Alzheimer's disease. This is an effect that we would not see for many years. It would also be a complete and utter disaster. I am not saying that this will happen, but I do think there is a real risk that it could. If you carry out major surgery on an important organ in the body, damaging its ability to function normally, you really need to be careful about what happens down the line.

Now, if we stuck to operating on the super-obese i.e. those with a body mass index greater than 45, or 50, the medical benefits are likely to far outweigh any potential downsides such as death, dementia and small bowel transplant – to name but three. However, it is clear that operations are being done on thinner and thinner people, for mainly cosmetic reasons, where it becomes far more likely that harm could significantly outweigh benefits.

At present, I drive past a poster every day which has a picture of a happy, smiling, attractive, and slim woman on it. It is advertising bariatric surgery at a local private hospital. The strapline suggests that bariatric surgery has utterly transformed her life, and made her a happy person. This is, essentially, cosmetic surgery and it is going to be paid for by relatively wealthy people – in most cases with no real health need.

Now I may be wrong about bariatric surgery and the harms that it may be found to cause. I have been wrong about things before. However, this procedure contains all of the elements that ring my alarm bells very loudly. I worry about the long-term effects. I worry about the lack of high quality evidence. I shall await confirmation one way, or another.

There are many other areas of medical management that it would be possible to look at in this chapter. However, going through them all would somewhat negate the purpose of what I have just written. Which is that is up to everyone to try to spot current activities that are likely to be found to be highly problematic in the future, ***and make up their own minds.***

Of course you cannot be 100% certain about any of this. However, you can ask yourself three questions which, I believe, may start you on the way:

- Does the idea seem very simple? Is it intuitive? Does it seem like common sense? (If so beware).

- How, and why, did it start being done? (Just because something is universally accepted as 'best practice', there is no reason to believe that it is beneficial).

- Ask yourself the key question. Was a randomised controlled study ever done before the activity first started? (Was, indeed, a study of any kind ever done?)

And always be happy with uncertainty. A thing can never be known for sure. We are always making best guesses, based on what we know today, and not tomorrow.

CHAPTER NINE

Never believe that something is impossible

"The mind likes a strange idea as little as the body likes a strange protein and resists it with similar energy. It would not perhaps be too fanciful to say that a new idea is the most quickly acting antigen known to science. If we watch ourselves honestly we shall often find that we have begun to argue against a new idea even before it has been completely stated."

Wilfred Trotter

"It was not noisy prejudice that caused the work of Mendel to lie dead for thirty years, but the sheer inability of contemporary opinion to distinguish between a new idea and nonsense."

Wilfred Trotter

I wrote this section mainly as a warning to everyone, including myself, to try to keep an open mind when reviewing ideas in medicine. I know that my ideas on cholesterol and heart disease are seen by many as completely whacko. When I say that a high cholesterol does not cause heart disease a lot of people roll their eyes and dismiss me before I have even had the chance to explain anything.

Such people just 'know' that cholesterol causes heart disease. They are as certain of this fact, as that the moon orbits the earth. It is common sense, it is known to be true, it fits in with our wider view of the world. Anyone who questions this has clearly lost touch with reality.

But the most dangerous possible way to think is to believe that something is *impossible*. To start dismissing a new idea before you have even started really listening to it. This is why my approach is to try to keep all ideas in one of three places. Probable, possible, or unlikely.

213

Could the earth go 'round the sun?

If you fall into the trap of absolutist thinking, that something is either right or wrong, true or false, good or bad, it becomes very difficult to change your mind. In significant part this is because, once we believe that we have successfully ascertained whether or not something is 'true' or 'false', we have built the solid foundations upon which we can build other ideas.

If, for example, we know that the sun goes round the earth, we can fit other observations around that. Over time we can create a more and more complex model of the solar system, with the Earth at the centre. It cannot work perfectly, of course, but it can nearly work so long as you are able to ignore such things as planets going in loops. (You can always call them paradoxical movements).

If you truly did sit down and think too hard about those loopy planets, the entire construction of the Geocentric (Earth at the middle) model would fall apart, and then what are you left with? Doubt, anxiety, uncertainty. Your world, and solar system, and understanding of the Universe has just been torn asunder. You have just obliterated a gigantic, interconnected belief structure that has taken hundreds of years, and thousands of people, to construct.

Ideas become closely woven together. They rely on each other, and our ideas are, to a great extent, what we are. We need them to make sense of the world around us. We hate them to be attacked.

"But I, being poor, have only my dreams; I have spread my dreams under your feet; Tread softly because you tread on my dreams."

W.B. Yeats

Another important reason why ideas persist with such stubborn resistance is the enormous difficulty of trying to get someone to see the world in a new way:

"When even the brightest mind in our world has been trained up from childhood in a superstition of any kind, it will never be possible for that mind, in its maturity, to examine sincerely, dispassionately, and conscientiously any evidence or any circumstance which shall seem to cast a doubt upon the validity of that superstition. I doubt if I could do it myself."

Mark Twain

I have often wondered what I would have believed if I had lived in Egypt 4,000 years ago. A bright shiny sphere would appear in the morning, drift across the sky and disappear at night, by definition I suppose. If someone had said to me, whilst we stood and watched the sunset, *'We are actually circling around that sun, not the other way around.'* How would I have reacted?

Me: *'Of course, how silly of me to think otherwise. It is so obvious. Thanks for putting me straight on that one... but, just one thing. What are we circling around in?'*

Not me: *'We are circling around in space.'*

Me: *'Space... of course. But what is space?'*

Not me: *'Space is nothing. It is emptiness.'*

Me: *'Right... So how do you know space is there? Also, how come we don't just fall. If the Earth is floating in space, shouldn't it fall down somewhere...'*

Not me: *'We cannot fall, because there is nowhere to fall to.'*

Me: *'Right... there is nowhere to fall to... So, let me try to get this straight. This massive Earth, the one I am standing on, is spinning around that very small sun in the sky, by floating through space – which doesn't exist. We don't fall, because there is nowhere to fall to... got it. One more thing, why do we rotate around the Sun, why don't we just fly off?'*

Not me: *'Because we are attracted to the sun by gravity, and thus remain within its orbit.'*

Me: *'Gravity, what's that?'*

Not me: *'Gravity is the force that attracts all matter towards other matter, and thus the Earth and the Sun are attracted to each other.'*

Me: *'Ok, can I see this gravity?'*

Not me: *'No, it is invisible. By the way the sun is far, far, larger than the Earth.'*

Me: *'Riiiight... Anyway, must be going, pyramid to build... Gods to placate.'*

Nowadays we just know that the Earth orbits around the Sun. It seems a simple and obvious thing to think. People who believe otherwise are mocked for their stupidity. But just try looking up at the sun, or the moon, and then try to wipe your mind clear of the last few hundred years of scientific thought and discovery.

What would you think? And what would you think of someone who came along and tried to explain how the solar system works. You would think, I suspect, that they were completely bonkers. Whilst we now know about gravity and space and orbits and suchlike, these are exceedingly complex ideas. Each one is mind-bogglingly difficult to accept. Also, importantly, we cannot see them. Which I think is also key to changing thinking.

Could the earth float around on tectonic plates?

When Wegener proposed his hypothesis that the surface of the Earth floated about on huge 'tectonic' plates, as this was clearly the best way to explain the structure of the continents, and continental drift, the main objections were that:

- The Earth's Geology can be fully explained by the 'Molten Earth' hypothesis. (The Earth got crinkly as it cooled down, forming mountains and oceans).

- You, Wegener, are not a geologist so you can know nothing of geology.

- How can huge plates 'float about' on the Earth's surface, how utterly ridiculous.

- Where are the joins between these plates, hmmmm? We cannot see any such thing.

The hypothesis of continental drift is a perfect example of how science rejects ideas. First, there was an existing hypothesis upon which eminent and learned experts had pinned their colours – and reputations. The cooling, crinkly, hypothesis. I think it has a posher name, so my son tells me, who is doing Geography, but that is exactly what it was.

There were then vicious personal attacks on Wegener, because he was not an 'expert' in the field of Geology. Ho hum. Then, of course, there was the apparent ridiculousness of the idea he was proposing 'The Earth's surface floats about... Really! And how does that happen... exactly!' Finally, and perhaps most importantly, the plates themselves could not be seen.

Or, to be more accurate, the joins between the plates could not be seen. Why not? Because they lie almost exclusively on the ocean floor.

They do appear above ground in some places, such as Iceland. And, once you know what you are looking at, you can see them clearly. You can also see them clearly in other places such as Scotland and the USA, and the Rift Valley. But when you do not wish to see what you are looking at, such things can be readily explained away as being something else. A big long valley for example.

It was not until the seabed started to be mapped by the US Navy that the joins between the plates became visible, stretching all around the world. At which point, suddenly, the hypothesis was accepted.

And so, we come to a vitally important issue that I feel has never really been discussed in the scientific literature. Well, it might have been, but I am unaware of such discussion. The issue is that we find it very difficult to believe in things we cannot see. Obviously you can quote many sayings *'Seeing is believing.' 'I will not believe until I have seen it with my own eyes.'* And suchlike.

I think these are more than just sayings. For most people the need to see a thing, really see it, is critical for acceptance. A great scientist may never need to physically see a thing, but they can visualise it. For most of the rest of us rather less gifted individuals, an image is a very powerful thing.

Could fat not clog arteries?

I firmly believe that one of the main reasons why the diet/heart cholesterol hypothesis grips the imagination so powerfully is that the images are so evocative. Here is a short section from a newspaper article:

> *"Photos taken inside clogged city sewer pipes look nearly identical to medical photos of the blood vessels of patients who have spent a lifetime gorging on fried chicken, sausage and bacon. 'It's like your arteries,' said John Parker, environmental compliance inspector with the city's Water and Sewer dept. 'Grease builds up in there. It's gory.'"*

Savannah Morning News

That is a strong and evocative image of stinky, fatty sludge, created by waste, and sloth. Surrounding that image, in most people's minds, will be mental pictures of fatty foods, slimy grease on plates, very fat people. Yuck.

The mind loves to create patterns and associations. In this case we have a 'gory' image of a sewage pipe, and this is associated with fried chicken, sausage and bacon. We now have a chain reaction going on, with thoughts of one thing triggering off a chain reaction of images. This creates an internal shudder of disgust. *'I am never going eat such horrible, fatty foods, ever again... ever.'* To which I can only say one thing. *'Bacon sandwich.'*

I remember Dr John Briffa remarking once. *"Why do people think that eating fat makes you fat. It must be word association."* I would say, nearly. I believe it is image and emotional association. Words, images and emotions become wrapped round each other in our brains.

In psychology this is called the 'Halo' effect. It is a hard-wired and primitive form of thought. Once we decide that something, or someone, is good. We see all of their actions in the light of this halo. This is a good person, e.g. Nelson Mandela, everything he does is good. This is a bad person e.g. Hitler, therefore everything they do is bad. We find it very hard to believe that good people can do bad things, and vice versa.

That is a slight detour from the power of pictures, and things we can see. Once we see a horrible image of fat in a sewer we can then build up a structure of thought around it. It is then but a short step to believe that all fat is disgusting, and that eating fat MUST therefore be bad for us. Nowadays, the Halo effect surrounding fat-avoidance has become very potent.

Watch a really fat person eating fatty food, and ask yourself how you feel. How you feel is why many really fat people eat only in private. All of this means that, when someone announces that fatty sludge builds up in your arteries, in much the same way it builds up in sewers, we find this idea sensible, straightforward and true. It fits with our internal images, emotions and prejudices. It just sounds right.

In fact the Halo effect with fat is so powerful that it underpinned a series of anti-smoking adverts in the UK. They showed fat dripping out of the end of cigarettes, instead of ash. It was a truly horrible image, with smokers leaving *streaks* of brown fat all over themselves.

The voiceover declared: *"Every cigarette we smoke makes this fatty stuff get stuck in our arteries. Our hearts can't work properly if our arteries are all clogged up."* Give up before you clog up was the message. I am perfectly sure that they tested out these images on various focus groups before deciding on the best message, and images. They will have found that pictures of fat were found to be *the* most disgusting and off-putting.

Of course it is the most ridiculous nonsense. Cigarettes may contain a lot of unhealthy substances, but one that they most definitely do not contain is fat. So how, exactly, can smoking a zero fat cigarette lead to the build-up of fat in your arteries? Answers on a post-card please – I am hoping to get a lot of post-cards!

Could hand washing save lives?

See it, believe it. Don't see it, don't believe it. Medicine has many examples of *'that which we cannot see, we deny.'* A perfect example of this would be the world of infectious diseases. Have you heard of a very great man called Semmelweis? No I thought not.

'Semmelweis suggested that it would be a good idea for doctors to wash their hands with chlorinated lime solutions. It was 1847 and he was working in Vienna General Hospital's First Obstetrical Clinic, where doctors' wards had three times the mortality of midwives' wards.

Despite published evidence where hand washing had reduced mortality to below 1%, Semmelweis's observations conflicted with the established scientific and medical opinions of the time and so his ideas were rejected. Some doctors were offended at the suggestion that they should wash their hands.

In 1865 Semmelweis was committed to an asylum, where he died at the age of 47. He was beaten by the guards within days of being committed. It wasn't until years after his death that Semmelweis was proven right. Louis Pasteur confirmed the germ theory and Joseph Lister, acting on the French microbiologist's research, practised and operated, using hygienic methods, with great success.

Ah, those jolly old eminent doctors again. *'How dare you tell us to wash our hands you bloody upstart. How can washing our hands with chlorinated lime solution possibly prevent infections and deaths. Hmmm. Gaze upon my splendid doctorly hands, you knave, can you see anything on them that could possibly cause women to die... thought not.'*

No wonder Semmelweis went mad.

At around about the same time John Snow, in London, effectively proved that cholera was a waterborne infection. He removed a pump handle in Broad Street and stopped an episode of cholera in its tracks.

This episode is presented to medical students as a kind of Hollywood moment where Snow, ridiculed for years, was finally carried through the street of London by a massive crowd, pump handle brandished above his head. The crowd reached the Houses of Parliament. *'God bless you Snow,'* a beautiful young woman cries, bosom heaving... *'you saved my little daughter's life.'* More wild cheering.

On the steps of Westminster, leading to the Mother of Parliaments, the Prime Minister meets Snow, bows stiffly, and declares *'Thank you for your work, John Snow, no-one shall ever die of Cholera again.'* Cue more wild cheering, fade to uplifting music. 'The motion picture was based on true events...' George Clooney (who else) played John Snow...

Is this what actually happened? Why, no, of course not. He, and his findings were dismissed as the ravings of a bloody upstart. *'Infectious agents, in water! Whomsoever could think such a blasted foolish thing.'*

I believe that he was dismissed, in major part, because no-one had ever seen an infectious agent in water, or anywhere else come to that:

"An outbreak of 20 cases (of cholera) on the hospital ship 'Dreadnought' in October 1837 was investigated by George Budd (brother of William Budd) and George Busk, who concluded aspects of the outbreak 'mitigate against the idea of its contagious nature'. Busk was a keen microscopist and examined cholera evacuations on the Dreadnought with negative findings."[127]

Can't see it, can't be there. Here are some of the eminent doctors of the time attacking John Snow. For being right, as it turns out.

"'There is, in our view, an entire failure of proof that the occurrence of any one case could be clearly and unambiguously assigned to water... Notwithstanding our opinion that Dr Snow has failed in proving that cholera is communicated in the mode in which he supposes it to be, he deserves the thanks of the profession for endeavouring to solve the mystery. It is only by close analysis of facts and the publication of new views that we can hope to arrive at the truth.' E.A. Parkes, a Professor of Hygiene in the Army Medical School, accused Snow of exaggeration."[128]

Yes, how cleverly they refuted John Snow. How smugly, how superiorly... how wrongly.

At the time, everyone knew that infections were spread by nasty smells. The 'Miasma' theory of infection. Quite amazingly, or at least I think it is amazing, a lengthy war between the British and the Dutch ended with the Dutch gaining control of the spice islands near Indonesia, in return for handing over New Amsterdam a.k.a. New York.

Yes indeed, when the dust settled over the Nutmeg Wars. The Dutch got the only two small islands in the world where nutmeg grew. Britain gained control of North America. A cracking bit of negotiation by the Brits for a change.

Why was nutmeg so valuable? Well it was known that the plague, as with any infection, was spread by smells/miasma. Put nutmeg into the vents in your plague mask and the smells go away. Which means that you can't get infected. Simple.

This is the ostrich approach to infection control. If you can't smell it, it can't get you. For the sake of this argument seeing and smelling are much the same thing. Can't see it, can't be there. Can't smell it, can't be there.

To give doctors of the time their due I suppose you can see where the Miasma theory came from. Unpleasant smells and infection definitely do go hand in hand. We can certainly smell rotting flesh and suchlike, even if we cannot see what is causing the smell, and eating rotten food makes you ill. Given this, you can see why the 'experts' of their time were certain that Miasma spread infection, not anything in water. Especially not anything so small that you could not even see it.

Could the body have a circulatory system?

This disbelief in things we can't see extends well beyond infection. Capillaries, for example. These are the extremely small blood vessels that link the arterial system to the venous system. When you can cut through a muscle you can see small arteries and small veins with the naked eye. However, you cannot see the capillaries that join them together because they are just too small.

Without anything to join them together, how could blood that flows down the arteries end up coming back through the veins? Magic? Or there had to be another explanation as to how the circulatory system worked. Actually it wasn't called the circulatory system at the time, because no-one believed that the blood actually circulated round the body.

Enter Galen, a doctor who lived in Roman times. He came up with a solution that, today, seems like the most complete nonsense. Galen believed that the circulatory system consisted of two separate one-way systems of distribution, rather than a single system of circulation. He thought that venous blood was generated in the liver, from where it was distributed and utilised by all organs of the body. He posited that arterial blood originated in the heart, from where it was distributed and utilised by all organs of the body.[129]

The liver made venous blood and the heart made arterial blood and the organs consumed it. Well, when you have two separate systems of blood vessels, arteries and veins, with no visible connection between the two – what solution would you come up with? It clearly made more sense than the idea that blood flowed down arteries and back up veins, with nothing to connect them.

Somewhat ironically, in order to make his system work better Galen also postulated that there were pores in the septum of the heart that allowed blood to transfer from the right side of the heart to the left side. For centuries doctors believed that they could see these invisible pores – even when they were not there. (Strange, you can believe in invisible pores in the heart, but not in the rest of the body – oh well).

Galen's views may not have been a major problem by themselves. After all, it was the type of mistake that any idiot could make. But Galen was such an enormously influential physician that to question his views was considered heresy by the Catholic Church, and you could easily find yourself executed for questioning him. He was *the* original, unquestionable, expert.

1,500 years later, or so, William Harvey figured out how the circulatory system worked. Actually, I would imagine a lot of people had figured out how the circulatory system worked before Harvey. I think the Arabs did it in about the ninth century. Harvey was just the first who published his ideas, and did not end up dangling on the end a rope.

"Although Harvey announced his discovery in 1615 he waited 13 years before publishing his results since it was considered sacrilegious to challenge Galen. Any contrary opinions were considered to be heretical, and would not only quickly end your career, but could even cause you to be burned at the stake.

"Harvey's hesitation to openly defy Galen proved to be justified. Most physicians rejected his 1628 book because he could not explain how the arteries and veins met. If organs did not consume blood, how did different parts of the body obtain nourishment? If the liver did not make blood from food, where did blood originate? Why was blood blue in veins but red in arteries? It took two decades for Harvey's colleagues to acknowledge his achievements." (From the American Newsletter on Stress 2008, volume 12.)

In this case it took the experts a mere two decades to accept the blindingly obvious! My, they were getting a move on in 1628. The seventeenth must have been a century of particular enlightenment.

Of course we all now know that Harvey was right, and how simple it seems. It always does after the event. I find it interesting that Harvey's observations were also accepted at just about the same time as other scientists, with their new-fangled microscopic devices, first noticed that there really were tiny little blood vessels that connected arteries to veins. Coincidental timing – possibly.

Don't mention autism!

Where, however, does this leave us today? Where are the modern day equivalents of things that cannot be seen and hypotheses that are currently dismissed as ridiculous because we do not have anything that we can see? If I were to bet, then one of the main areas would be in the area of mitochondrial dysfunction, including Chronic Fatigue Syndrome and – horror of horrors – vaccine damage.

Whilst you can certainly see mitochondria with a big microscope, it is exceedingly difficult to measure their energy production. I have read many papers on this subject and it seems that, although there are ways to do this, it is complicated and the results are far from certain. However, if the mitochondria in your cells are not working properly then you are knackered – literally and metaphorically, and you can become very unwell indeed.

At this point, for those of you who consider vaccination to be the most wonderful thing, with no downsides whatsoever, please look away now...

Virtually no doctor in Britain is aware that a young girl called Hannah Polling in the USA was awarded massive damages for the finding that her autism was 'caused' by childhood vaccination. $13,000,000 in damages, I believe.

Why were damages awarded? Because it was accepted that she had underlying mitochondrial dysfunction. This was worsened by vaccination, leading to autism spectrum disorder (ASD).

In fact, that is not quite accurate. The judgement was distinctly... weird. So tortured did the language become in this case that I thought I should reproduce part of a press report:

"Officials at the US Department of Health and Human Services investigating Hannah's medical history said that vaccines had 'significantly aggravated an underlying mitochondrial disorder, which predisposed her to deficits in energy metabolism', causing damage 'with features of autism spectrum disorder'. The officials said that the vaccine didn't 'cause' her autism, but 'resulted' in it."[130]

The vaccine didn't cause her autism, but resulted in it. Try to pick the grammar out of that one... The vaccine "resulted" in her autism? I have tried every version of this, in all directions, and I cannot make any sense of it at all. Oh well, when you are trying to twist reality through 180 degrees, language ends up strangled to death and gasping its last breath on the floor.

At this point I have to make a disclaimer. I am aware that to breathe the slightest possibility that vaccination may cause autism is the medical equivalent of blasphemy. To dare to do so, is to be cast into the ninth layer of medical hell. So I would just like to take the opportunity to state that, in general, I am greatly pro-vaccination. Indeed, I consider vaccination against many diseases to be one of the greatest of all medical achievements.

However, I do *not* think this means that discussion and debate is, therefore, irresponsible and impossible. My personal view of debate is that it is something I engage in to learn. When did debate become dangerous and forbidden? Every doctor knows the unspoken rule in this world now, which is that you cannot ever criticise any aspect of vaccination. It is made very clear that the moment you do this, you will instantly be accused of causing parents to stop vaccinating their children, and therefore millions will die blah, blah... blah.

Well then, what should we make of this?

"An increased risk of narcolepsy was found following vaccination with Pandemrix, a monovalent 2009 H1N1 influenza vaccine that was used in several European countries during the H1N1 influenza pandemic. Narcolepsy is a chronic neurological disorder caused by the brain's inability to regulate sleep-wake cycles normally. This risk was initially found in Finland, and then some other European countries also detected an association. Most recently, scientists at the United Kingdom's (UK) Health Protection Agency (HPA) have found evidence of an association between Pandemrix and narcolepsy in children in England. The findings are consistent with studies from Finland and other countries."[131]

Oh, look, more vaccine damage. Guess what the underlying problem is thought to be in narcolepsy. Yup, mitochondrial dysfunction. As regards the fact that vaccines cannot possibly damage you, as far back as 1979 a vaccine damage act was passed in the UK. Bet you didn't know that.

"An Act to provide for payments to be made out of public funds in cases where severe disablement occurs as a result of vaccination against certain diseases or of contact with a person who has been vaccinated against any of those diseases; to make provision in connection with similar payments made before the passing of this Act; and for purposes connected therewith."

224

Blah, blah...

The US has one of these acts too. Now, why would you pass an Act in Parliament, or Congress, to provide payments for severe 'disablement' as a result of vaccine damage? Would this be because vaccine damage never occurs? Or that it occurs quite often? Or occurs at all? Hmmmm, let me think.

In truth, the figures on vaccine damage are exceedingly difficult to analyse, because causality is very difficult to prove on a case by case basis. However, when it comes to negative findings I always like to go to Germany. It has been demonstrated many times that the Germans are the most likely to report negative findings accurately. Yes I know, terrible racial stereotyping, but a fact is a fact. What do the Germans have to say on the matter?

"Between 1978 and 1993 approx. 13,500 cases of undesired effects resulting from medications for vaccinations was reported to the Paul Ehrlich-Institute (PEI) which is the institute which is responsible for vaccine security; the majority was reported by the pharmaceutical industry. In 40% of these cases the complications were severe, 10% pertained to fatalities on account of effects."[132]

5,400 severe complications, and a 10% fatality rate. This, as you may have worked out for yourself, represents 1,350 deaths, or about 100 per year. Remember that these are only the absolutely, rigorously, confirmed deaths due to vaccination. There could have been far more, there could *not* have been less.

The Germans have updated their vaccine damage system since that first report from the years 1978 to 1993:

Since early 2001 the federal infection protection law now mandates that severe cases are reported directly to the PEI immediately after the vaccination. These are listed as follows...

"Potential severe reactions/follow-up damages after vaccinations:

- *Chronic immune weakness involving frequent infections (frequently repeatedly inner ear infections)*

- *Encephalopathia = brain disease (This is a brain edema caused by the vaccination; it mainly pertains to children younger than 3 years of age who cannot react to the vaccination with an infection because their brains are not yet fully developed). Encephalopathia is frequently overlooked as it does not always entail severe symptoms. However, there can later be developmental retardation. Encephalopathia can also trigger cri encéphalique.*

- *Screaming/Cri encéphalique (usually extremely penetrating and shrill) = sign of potential brain damage*

- *Autoimmune diseases (please refer also to vaccinations and immune system)*

- *Trigger of allergies such as asthma, skin allergies, hay fever, food allergies... (please refer also to vaccinations and immune system)*

- *Seizures*

- *Epilepsia*

- *Autism*

- *Sleeping sickness*

- *Sleep reversal (child awake and restless at night, sleeps during the day)*

- *Personality changes, behavioral disorders, difficult to train, hyperactive children, ADS, apathy*

- *Diabetes*

- *Multiple sclerosis*

- *Delay of development of language*

- *SID (Sudden infant death)"*

"A large number of the vaccine reactions and vaccine damages are being discussed presently. There are controversies pertaining to particularly diabetes, autism and multiple sclerosis, i.e. whether there is a connection between these diseases and vaccinations? It is always problematic to 'prove' damages as they frequently do not occur until months later and thus a causal connection can be negated."[132]

An interesting little list of things here, including: immune weakness, seizures, brain disease, epilepsy and death. Also, autism... well, well, who'd a thunk.

I am more than acutely aware that there is an extraordinarily paternalistic point of view when it comes to vaccination. *'Not in front of the children. We must tell everyone that vaccination is a universal good and no questioning can possibly be allowed. Look what happened with Andrew Wakefield and MMR etc.'*

Well, in my opinion the response of those in power to Andrew Wakefield just made the situation far, far, worse. The correct response to his research, and the following overblown pronouncements, should have been something along the lines of. '*We are aware of his research and we are looking at it closely. It has understandably created concerns with many parents. We do not believe that there is any link between the MMR vaccine and autism, but we are studying his research closely to make certain...*'

There, wouldn't that have been nice? Nice and scientific, and responsible.

Instead the approach was to attack him personally, along with all of those associated with him. Take them to court, threaten to throw them in jail, remove their license to practise medicine etc. This had the exact effect that you would expect.

It made many people feel that Wakefield was probably onto something, and that the Government was covering things up. For many, Wakefield is now seen as a brave heroic figure, battling corrupt big pharma and Governments around the world.

My own frustration is that you cannot now even attempt to discuss what he may have found, at all, anywhere, ever. This whole area is just shut off completely. Dare to mention even the teeniest thing that Wakefield said, and it is made crystal clear that you, too, will suffer his fate.

At one time I wrote a column for *Pulse* magazine in the UK, which is the best read magazine for UK General Practitioners. Most of it was vaguely controversial. Cancer screening is a waste of time. Don't take statins... That type of thing. I could say pretty much what I liked. But when I wrote an article criticising the demonising of Wakefield, they just would not publish it.

I did not say that MMR caused autism. I did not say that Wakefield was correct. I just objected to the way he was personally attacked and vilified. I opined that this was not the way to have any sort of debate on such an important issue. My view was that he could be a corrupt and unpleasant individual – but he could still be right. His personality had no bearing on the science. I have no idea of his morals, or personality.

However, this is not the position taken up by most people, or indeed most doctors. Here, for example, is a comment on Wakefield, published on a doctor's forum in the UK

"*Considering he violated the Geneva accords for research, perforated the colon of a child doing an unethical, unconsented, non-indicated colonoscopy, and published fraudulently – why is he not somewhere hot, chained at the ankle, breaking rocks?*"

Here is another one

"I do wish Wakefield would just #### off. I really do."

And another

"The arrogance of Wakefield and his deluded 'supporters' astounds me. It is a pity that criminal charges cannot be brought against this charlatan."

I could fill a book with quotes like this. However, I have already covered the issue of nasty, vindictive, personal attacks on scientists saying things the mainstream does not like, and why this should have no place in scientific discussions. However, because of Wakefield, the entire area of vaccine damage has been placed behind police security tape with '*no entry*' signs fluttering in the breeze.

I believe that this is a massive problem. For if it turns out that mitochondrial dysfunction makes some children, or adults, susceptible to vaccine damage, then we might be able to research this phenomenon, and prevent it... IF PEOPLE WERE ALLOWED TO RESEARCH THIS AREA WITHOUT BEING VICIOUSLY ATTACKED. Sorry to shout, but this whole area makes me somewhat angry.

We already know that around 100 children die in Germany each year from severe reaction to vaccination. I don't even like to calculate what this adds up to worldwide. So this is not some minute and abstract risk. Wouldn't it be nice to be able to study why this might be happening, in an attempt to stop it? Why yes, of course it would. Anyone like to make it a research project... anyone... thought not.

Don't mention ME either

To further develop the main issue here, which is mitochondrial dysfunction. Of course, on one hand, it is well accepted amongst the scientific community that mitochondrial dysfunction exists. Some people believe it could be the underlying cause of Chronic Fatigue Syndrome (CFS) and/or Myalgic Encephalomyelitis (ME).

I can just see any doctor – who may have got this far in the book – hurling it across the room at this point. Not only does Kendrick believe that we should look into the possibility that vaccination might damage some people, but he has now dared to mention the most irritating of medical conditions, Chronic Fatigue Syndrome.

Nothing, and I mean nothing, causes more scathing commentary amongst the medical profession than ME/CFS. I started a discussion thread on ME/CFS on a doctors forum, suggesting that it may have an organic basis. I quoted what I thought was some quite reasonable research. There was little support, from anyone. Actually it would be more accurate to say that there was no support, anywhere, from anyone.

I stated:

"Not the slightest hint from anyone, so far, that they may open their minds just the tiniest crack to allow the possibility that CFS may have a real, organic, cause."

I wonder why not?

This was followed by another doctor who copied my post, and added their own comment:

"Not the slightest hint from anyone, so far, that they may open their minds just the tiniest crack to allow the possibility that CFS may have a real, organic, cause."

Because every single patient with 'ME' I have ever met has been a neurotic layabout.

Other comments followed, including this one:

"The term Myalgic encephalomyelitis gives a spurious scientific flavour to this phenomenon. Chronic Fatigue Syndrome, which is tending to replace ME, at least does not pre-suppose a biological process.

"However the abbreviation ME as in Me, me, me does in my opinion sum up the majority of sufferers who combine self-obsession with anger against the world in general and doctors in particular. I have never understood how people who are so fatigued can nevertheless run an ME society which is so active and aggressive in its attacks on anyone who questions ME that it has effectively shut down debate about the condition in the media and got the government to agree to make it a disability."

Etc.

Now, it could be that ME/CFS is purely a psychological condition suffered by *'neurotic layabouts.'* Indeed, I suspect that the ME/CFS card is played by some people for their own complex reasons. However, when Clare Francis, a woman who can sail single-handed across the Atlantic then finds that she can barely move, surely our minds should be open?

Perhaps no organic cause will ever be found, but I doubt it. I doubt it because we have at least one condition that used to be written off as CFS, but now, a true organic cause has been found. It is Lyme disease.

Lyme disease encompasses all the signs and symptoms of CFS, but doctors are now happy to call it something else, because an infective agent can be seen. A spirochete bacteria called *Borrelia burgdorferi.*

This bacterium gets into your body, primarily, through a tick bite. It then hides inside cells, as infective agents are wont to do. The primary problem in Lyme disease, which may be a spectrum of different diseases, is *damage to the mitochondria*, resulting in greatly decreased energy output. Yes it those pesky little mitochondria again.

With Lyme disease we have a condition that doctors love. It is difficult to diagnose, thus making the diagnosis itself an heroic act. The patient is also exceedingly grateful – having been routinely dismissed for being a neurotic layabout by other doctors. Once diagnosed, there is also a cure, which is the icing on the cake.

However, the point I am trying to make here is that, once we have managed to find a cause for CFS, it is no longer CFS, it is Lyme Disease. Yet, if someone has exactly the same symptoms and we cannot see a cause, the patient is often dismissed as a malingerer with ME, me, me, me. *'We can't find anything wrong, you can't have anything wrong with you, you, you are just making it up.'*

Could it possibly be that another infectious agent – that we cannot currently see, or recognise, could also cause other cases or CFS? Or could other things that we don't yet even know about cause mitochondrial dysfunction? Heavy metals, mercury, other toxins, trans-fats, stress? Yes, of course it is possible, but because we have no tests, no diagnosis, we write it off.

In large part we write it off because, not only can we not see an underlying cause. We cannot spot any measurable abnormality. People say they have no energy, but we do not measure this. Or, to be more accurate, we do not bother to measure this, because it is costly and complex.

There is, however, one group of researchers who have tried to measure mitochondrial function in ME/CFS. They took blood samples from people with the symptoms of ME/CFS and measured the function of mitochondria in white blood cells. This correlates reasonably, if not perfectly, with mitochondrial function throughout the body.

In their own words, when looking at people complaining of ME/CFS:

"We find that all patients tested have measureable mitochondrial dysfunction which correlates with the severity of the illness."[133]

Now you would think that this would be a pretty hot area of research. However if you look up ME/CFS and mitochondria in PubMed, the database of almost all published medical research, at the time of writing, you find a very lonely three citations. One of which is just a letter, not even a research paper.

So, in the entire world of medical research, we have two studies on the measurement of mitochondrial dysfunction in ME/CFS. Therefore, if I were to tell you that this is a veritable hot-bed of mainstream research, this would not be entirely accurate.

And for those of you who may take the time to look up this reference, and who thought that the name of one of the authors rings a few bells, you're right. It is Sarah Myhill. Another modern day medical pariah. Not quite in the Duesberg and Wakefield league, but maybe top of the championship, trying hard for promotion to premier league.

She has been hauled in front of the General Medical Committee (GMC), the organisation that disciplines doctors in the UK, where she was severely censured and punished over the content of her website, and her medical practice. As reported a couple of years ago:

Dr Myhill is now forbidden from prescribing any prescription-only medication and has been ordered to remove from her website content relating to the following:

- The medical management of cases relating to cardiology, or cardiovascular disease including; chest pain due to ischaemic heart disease; acute coronary syndrome; heart failure; or pulmonary embolus;

- The treatment of asthma;

- The treatment, testing, identification, diagnosis or management of breast cancer;

- The use of hormonal contraceptive medication;

- The pharmacological management of primary or secondary prevention of vascular disease;

- Any immunisation or vaccination.

They have also placed a range of restrictions on her with regard to seeking employment.[134]

By golly, in what seems like endlessly repeating pattern, her major crime was to suggest that vaccination may cause ME/CFS, or even autism, in some people. The very thing Hannah Polling received $13m for in the USA. Having committed this unforgivable sin, Sarah Myhill is now languishing in the Andrew Wakefield zone 'He-who-must-not-be-named.' Or in Myhill's case 'She-who-must-not-be-named.'

What is it about the area of viruses and vaccines, that becoming involved with either area creates such incandescent heat and rage. As mentioned a few times, there are two things you absolutely cannot say in medicine:

- Vaccines can cause damage, maybe even brain damage – perhaps even autism;

- HIV may not be the cause of AIDS.

It is impossible to discuss these issues, or debate them. If you stray into these topics you take your life into your hands. *'Trespassers will be subject to deadly force.'*

Unfortunately, because of the close connections between ME/CFS, mitochondrial dysfunction, and potential vaccine damage, anyone interested in studying ME/CFS will be, as with vaccines, frightened off. It is already viewed as a career limiting choice.

PhD Student: *'I would like to look into the area of mitochondrial function and ME/CFS.'*

Professor: *'Indeed, ho, ho. Study, the benefits of statins instead young man.'*

PhD student: *'But there are already 32,687 papers in this area, and counting.'*

Professor: *'Good grief, you can never have enough papers about statins. So get to it... pip, pip. There's a good chap. As for ME/CFS, **not** in my dept young fellow.'*

The next big thing

Through the centuries, medicine has been instantly ready to dismiss things that cannot (yet) be seen. Capillaries, microbes, microbes in the gut (H Pylori), and most recently, mitochondrial dysfunction. And just to take a quick detour into my pet subject, statins.

Statins cause muscle damage in many people. Mainstream medical thinking is that you measure creatinine kinase (CK) to see if muscle pain is due to statin damage (CK is an enzyme found in muscle cells, and leaks out into the bloodstream if muscle cells are damaged). It is generally accepted that if you do not have raised CK levels, there is no real damage and nothing to worry about. Certainly nothing to do with statins.

However, it has been proven repeatedly that severe muscle damage can occur without CK levels going up.

"Boston, MA – Persistent muscle pain in patients taking statins reflects structural muscle damage, and this microscopic damage can occur in the absence of elevated creatine phosphokinase levels, according to the results of a new study.

"'It's clear that a patient with statin-induced myopathy can have microscopic muscle damage, but the damage is not sufficient to break the cell open, and that means that it doesn't release creatinine phosphokinase into the blood,' said study investigator Dr Richard Karas (Tufts-New England Medical Center, Boston, MA). 'So to say that the other way around, we have clear evidence that there is ongoing damage to the muscle at the microscopic level, but it's not revealed in the blood tests that we use to check for muscle damage.'"[135]

Has this research made the slightest difference to anything? No. If a patient, on a statin, says they have muscle pain, the doctor may measure CK levels. Or, more likely the patient reporting adverse effects will just be dismissed. If CK is not raised, the doctor tells the patient that it is not the statin causing the muscle pain. Can't see it, can't be there.

In management circles it is often stated 'that which gets measured, gets managed.' In medicine, I am afraid to say *'that which cannot be measured, or seen, gets ignored.'* Or filed under... neurotic layabout.

I must say that I am fully guilty of this myself. As a doctor there is nothing more satisfying that finding something *'wrong.'* A raised or lowered level in the blood, or a lump. If something is raised, and then you can lower it, even better. If a lump can be removed... great. If it is a cancerous lump... double, super, great.

Yes, as a profession we are extra sympathetic to cancer. It is real, it is very serious, and we feel nothing but sympathy for the patient. I work near Christie's hospital in Manchester and the care and compassion that patients receive there is amazing. Everyone goes the extra mile, and nothing is too much.

But I would argue that cancer is emotionally easy to connect with. It is the most real of real diseases. It is serious, it is proper medicine, it can be scanned and monitored and measured, and we can all place ourselves in the shoes of those suffering from it. People wear badges and go on sponsored walks, and set up charities for cancer. Try organising an ME/CFS walk. Yes, I know, you won't get very far... ho, ho.

233

On the other hand, nothing is more energy sapping than having to deal with patients with a problem that cannot be seen, measured, or lowered, or removed, or treated in some way. For example TATT. A large proportion of all GP consultations are for TATT. There are specific blood tests for TATT, and if you write TATT on the request form, a series of tests will be done. And what, you may ask, is TATT.

It stands for Tired All The Time (TATT). *'I don't know what is wrong with me doctor, I just feel tired all the time.'* I just can't tell you the sense of deep joy that this opening gambit fills a doctor with. Maybe because, despite what my family tell me, I am actually very empathetic. Because, when someone tells me they feel tired all the time, it also makes me feel very, very, tired. My head droops, and my enthusiasm for life burns a little less brightly. I become aware of the clock ticking on the wall – time slows...

Of course TATT is not really the correct diagnosis anymore. It is TATTS. Tired All The Time Syndrome. What is it about the word syndrome that provides authenticity? As with loud and out of control children who could, in earlier times, be described as annoying little brats. They now have oppositional syndrome. They certainly fill me with UCVS (Urge to Commit Violence Syndrome).

Of course, the first step with TATTS is easy. Send them for a series of blood tests to look for a variety of – accepted – causes of tiredness. Anaemia, Hypothyroidism, Diabetes and such like. In about 99.99999999999% of cases, no cause is found. All tests come back normal.

Then what?

Whilst many of these people are probably stressed, or mildly depressed, what of the others? They cannot all be stressed, or depressed. So, unless you are willing to write off vast numbers of patients as malingering layabouts, something must be going on.

Because many doctors obviously share my body language when confronted by someone with TATTS, patients get fed up with mainstream medicine and drift over to look at homeopathy, and crystallotherapy, and kerlian photography – whatever that may actually be. When they visit those offering such services, they are usually told that they have a deficiency of this, that, or the other thing. Then they need fifty courses of that thing – at fifty pounds a pop. Which is a side issue.

What is most important here is that many people do not have enough energy. In fact, I would say that a lack of energy is one of the most important health problems that there is. In that it affects the quality of life of many, many, people. Yet we *never* measure energy production. Never ever, ever... ever.

We measure blood pressure, and cholesterol levels, and thyroid levels, and liver and kidney function. We have MRI scanners and CT scanners and PET scans, and uncle Tom Cobbly and all. We spend billions measuring various bits of human physiology, but we have chosen not to measure energy production.

This is strange, because energy is all that we are really. Almost all of our organs are either involved in producing it, or using it. They have no other real function. We eat to provide energy. Our GI system, including the liver, converts what we eat into small molecules that can, when acted on by enzymes, produce energy.

The brain and muscles use energy, the kidneys get rid of the waste molecules of energy production. Our lungs suck in oxygen, required to run energy production in our cells. We are creatures of energy, and yet we study everything but. Mainstream medicine seems absurdly disinterested as to how energy production in cells can be measured and, hopefully, improved.

Could it be, just possibly, that energy dysfunction, or whatever term you feel most comfortable with, is at the heart of many 'illnesses'? Could it be, for example, that if you manipulate energy fields around, say, a broken bone, then the bone might heal more rapidly? Well, whether you believe it or not – it works. Pulsed Electromagnetic Therapy is now pretty well established as a technique to improve bone healing, healing of other damaged tissues, and it also works in depression. Could it also be that electromagnetic fields can be used to treat migraines? Why, yes, it can.

Most doctors still make that strangely effective harrumphing noise of contempt when such things are discussed. 'Oh, you believe in that... reeeeaaally.' Danger, nutcase alert. Whoop, whoop! I just gaze at them and wonder at their perfect certainty that everything that can be known, is known.

I am oft reminded of Lord Kelvin who is reported, famously, to have announced at the Royal Society at the end of the nineteenth century that... *"There is nothing new to be discovered in physics now. All that remains is more and more precise measurement."* Well, quite. I assume the first atomic bomb would have come as a bit of a shocker to him, had he still been alive. As for x-rays, the space time continuum and quantum theory... and suchlike... least said, soonest mended.

I think if I were forced to make one prediction upon which to rest my reputation, it would be that diseases of energy production/dysfunction will turn out to be the next great field of medical discovery and research.

Also, and most importantly, if you want to look into medical research and decide if it is important, or nonsense, do not dismiss those who appear to be talking nonsense. Do not dismiss ideas as 'impossible'. It was considered impossible that bacteria could live in the human stomach – so Groves and Warren were dismissed by the 'experts'. Until, that is, they won the Nobel Prize.

John Snow was dismissed, Semmelweiss was dismissed, Wegener was dismissed, Galileo was dismissed. We should all be very wary of dismissing anything. This form of thinking is, what is now called, system 1 thinking. When you start thinking about medicine, please engage system 2 thinking.

It is Daniel Kahneman who has best analysed the differences between system 1 and system 2 thinking. I mentioned him earlier. He is brilliant, even though I entirely absolutely and totally disagree with his assertion that we have to believe in the experts. As you may have picked up already, this book is, at heart, a 100,000 word plea to think for yourself, and constantly question the 'experts'.

Here is a good summary of Kahneman's ideas on different types of thinking:

Kahneman is a researcher and his descriptions of the results of years of testing people is fascinating... he divides most thinking into two parts: "Fast" or more intuitive thinking which he calls System 1 and "Slow" or more rational thinking which he calls System 2. These are two ways of interpreting the world around us based on the facts we perceive or let ourselves perceive. System 1 wants to fit what it sees into a pattern as quickly as possible so it can assess the threat level of what's happening. System 2 wants to take its time to evaluate rationally the input it receives. The problem comes when System 1 decides too quickly and System 2, which is prone to laziness, just agrees. There are a number of tests or riddles he uses that illustrate this. My favourite: a bat and a ball cost $1.10, the bat costs $1 more than the ball, how much does the ball cost? What do you think? Read the book for the answer! (It's not ten cents!)

In my view, medicine is hamstrung by far too much system 1 thinking.

CHAPTER TEN

'Facts' can be, and often are, plucked from thin air

"The great enemy of the truth is very often not the lie – deliberate, contrived and dishonest, but the myth – persistent, persuasive, and unrealistic. Belief in myths allows the comfort of opinion without the discomfort of thought."

John F. Kennedy

Of all the things that I write about, and lecture about, and talk about, and pontificate about, the thing that people always appear to have the greatest difficult accepting is when I tell them that the 'fact' they have heard a thousand times, was just made up. Or, to put it another way was 'plucked from thin air.'

Earlier on in the book I discussed the process by which this happens, but I think it is worth repeating this critical point again. So, pay attention. Many medical facts are not facts in any sense of the word, they have simply been made up. And that, ladies and gentlemen, is a fact.

When I worked with the European Society of Cardiology to help develop educational materials, one of the things we were very keen to do was to try to find the supporting evidence behind 'best medical practice.'

When we looked for evidence we were trying to use 'evidence', and not just 'evidence.' It may surprise you, or maybe not, that medical evidence comes in at least six different strengths. Ranging from a systemic review of randomised controlled trails, all the way down to expert opinion, the lowest form of human... evidence.

If you have read to this point, I suppose it will come as no surprise to find that, in the vast majority of cases, around 80%, the evidence used was the lowest level. Level IV, otherwise known as 'expert committee reports, opinion and/or clinical experience of respected authorities'. This would otherwise be known as medicine based on anecdote by important professors. Or, as one wag has put it, this is *'Eminence based medicine.'* Or *'Do you know who the bloody hell I am, medicine.'*

Essentially, most of accepted medical practice is, rather frighteningly, based on nothing other than someone's opinion, or subjective observations. Even more frighteningly, in my opinion, medical practice that is considered to be of the highest quality e.g. Ia 'practice based on randomised controlled trials' rests almost entirely on clinical trials funded and run by the pharmaceutical industry. We have already seen how free from bias such evidence can be.

I say frighteningly, because if this evidence is wrong, biased, or corrupted, the effects can be absolutely catastrophic. I wrote a blog on the topic of the damage done by one set of purportedly evidence based guidelines that were based on research that turned out to be falsified.

From a blog written in January 2014:[137]

Guidelines kill 800,000

A few days ago a friend sent me this headline by e-mail.

"Guideline Based on Discredited Research May Have Caused 800,000 Deaths In Europe Over The Last 5 Years."

i would replace the word *'May'* with these two words *'almost certainly.'* You would think, would you not, that if any other event in the world, at any time, had killed 800,000 people, this would be front page headlines around the world for weeks, probably months, maybe even years.

238

Governments would spring into action, those guilty dragged into court. Thousands would protest in the streets, petitions would be signed, laws passed.

The reality is, I am willing to bet, that you have never even heard of this gigantic scandal. It will not have appeared in any national television programme, or newspaper. The blogosphere is also, almost totally silent.

Eight hundred thousand people. Please let that figure sink in for a few moments. If you dropped a major thermonuclear device on Manchester (UK) and killed every single living person, this would be roughly equivalent. If you laid the corpses end to end, the line of dead people would stretch from John O Groats to Land's End (the entire length of the UK). Walking briskly each day, it would take you two months to pass them.

Think on that.

To an extent the actual guidelines themselves are not the most important thing here. They are now in the process of being changed (although they have not yet been changed). Nobody can be brought back to life, those who could have died – are dead. The issue here is that the processes leading to the creation of guidelines, which have almost certainly killed 800,000 people, are still in place, with no prospect of any change.

Those who have read this blog may be aware of my distaste for medical guidelines, and my concerns about their impact. I wrote an earlier blog called "Who shall guard the guardians?" This outlined some of the problems, but even I was overwhelmed by the sheer scale of deaths involved when guidelines go wrong. I could have worked it out, but never did.

Guidelines are based on evidence, and evidence is based on clinical trials. And major clinical trials are, almost without exception, paid for, run, and controlled by the pharmaceutical industry. The great and good of medicine, the 'Key Opinion Leaders' KOLs, who put together the guidelines will almost all have very close connections with the industry. In some cases they will have been paid significant amounts of money by pharmaceutical companies, although the Sunshine Act may start to put a block on this.

Whether they think so, or not, these opinion leaders are biased. Biased in favour of pharmaceutical products that are promoted through biased research, and launched on an unsuspecting world. And there is no one out there to check what these KOLs and guideline committees are doing. If, to pluck a name from the air, the European Society of Cardiology (ESC) decides to create a guideline committee, how do they do it?

239

They choose a chairman, who will be on one of their committees. A well regarded, sound chap, with expertise in the area. He, very rarely she, will then decide on which of his friends and colleagues would be most suitable to be committee members.

They will have a few meetings, gather the evidence together, decide on what best practice should be, and produce their guidelines. No other organisation checks on them, or their decision making, or their conflicts of interest. Or, indeed, the evidence itself.

Yet, when the guidelines come out, many countries will slavishly follow them. They will form the basis for instructions to their medical services. Doctors who fail to follow the guidelines can be censured, or lose their jobs. They virtually carry the force of law.

Something this powerful and important and critical to medical care is dealt with in an almost completely cavalier fashion. Which is, frankly, inexcusable.

I suppose you are wondering what these guidelines were? Well, they were on the use of beta-blockers to protect the heart during surgery. To see more on this story go to the Forbes website.[138]

I cannot send you to the article published in the *European Heart Journal*, because one hour after going up on their website, it was pulled. Here is the comment from the authors of this paper, Graham Cole and Darrel Francis, on the decision of the Editor to disappear the article.

"Our article is a narrative of events with a timeline figure and a context figure. We had not considered it to contain scientific statements, but we admit that it does multiply together three published numbers.

"It is not an analysis of individual trials considering design, molecule, dose and regimen. We published last year the formal meta-analysis under stringent peer review in Heart and addressed the questions, including dosing, in that paper and associated correspondence.

"The first of our two EHJ articles merely says that our community, which races to take credit when research-led therapy improves survival, must be equally attentive to the possibility of harm. The leverage of leadership means the magnitude of either may be far from trivial.

"Where our article relayed numbers, we made clear that alternative values were possible. The focus for readers was on how serious the consequences can be when clinical research goes wrong.

"We thank Prof Lüscher for highlighting the scientifically important point that the pivotal trial, DECREASE I, has not been retracted by NEJM because the

investigative committee did not recommend this. Unfortunately the committee could not have done so, because DECREASE I was outside its brief, displayed on the first text page of the first committee report. Can readers suggest why DE-CREASE I, from the same trial family, was exempted from inquiry?

"We admire Prof Lüscher's diligence in sending for peer review what we thought was merely multiplication. We await the review of the pair of articles. The first narrated one instance of a pervasive problem. The second suggests what each of us can do to reduce recurrences.

"We respect the process Prof Lüscher has set in motion. We ask readers to join with us, and the journal, in maximizing the reliability of clinical science for the benefit of patients."

Well, I am really glad that this article is being sent for peer review, because – as we know – peer review is a jolly good thing. Please forgive me for repeating this quotation from Richard Horton, Editor of *The Lancet*, but it is so apt in more than one place in this book:

"The mistake, of course, is to have thought that peer review was any more than a crude means of discovering the acceptability — not the validity — of a new finding. Editors and scientists alike insist on the pivotal importance of peer review. We portray peer review to the public as a quasi-sacred process that helps to make science our most objective truth teller. But we know that the system of peer review is biased, unjust, unaccountable, incomplete, easily fixed, often insulting, usually ignorant, occasionally foolish, and frequently wrong."

Frankly, I wouldn't hold my breath waiting for peer review on this matter.

I suppose you may also be wondering how the problem with these guidelines came to light. Well, it turns out that the chairman of the guidelines committee was Prof Don Poldermans. A man who has now been booted out of his job at Erasmus Hospital in the Netherlands for making up his research. The very research that was used to create these guidelines.

Don Poldermans also had financial conflicts of interest with Merck, Pfizer, Novartis and Medtronic. To name but four. (One conflict of interest statement can be seen here).[139]

Anyway, here is a summary of what happened:

- Don Poldermans had financial conflicts of interest with several pharmaceutical companies;

- Don Poldermans carried out corrupt research, supporting the use of pharmaceutical products;

- Don Poldermans was the chairman of an ESC (European Society of Cardiology) committee that recommended widespread use of drugs to protect the heart during surgery;

- An article reporting the widespread use of drugs to protect the heart during surgery suggested that they had killed 800,000 people over 5 years in Europe (alone);

- The paper outlining the scale of deaths has been pulled by the ESC.

I hope the hell there are no more Don Poldermans out there... but you would have to be a brave man to think so. Personally, I believe there is an endemic problem with bias and corruption in medical research, and we should be very afraid indeed...

It is said that when medical students start medical school they are all still told that... '*50% of what we are teaching you is wrong. We just don't know which 50%.*' I haven't actually checked if this is true, or not. But enough people have said it... so I suspect it is probably a myth.

If it is not true however, then it damned well should be. However, I would change the statement somewhat. '*Dear medical student. About 80% of what you are about to be taught is based on no clinical evidence whatsoever. Of the rest, about 50% is so biased that you should ignore it. Of the remaining 10%, about 50% will be proven to be wrong in the future.*'

Too drastic a statement. Well, in one way this is true, much of what is taught to medical students is obviously correct. Human anatomy, physiology, biochemistry, pathophysiology, the vast majority of this stuff is true, and it is unlikely to change. New things will be discovered, but it will build onto what we know, rather than tear it down.

Many medical interventions are also 'true' and will remain so. Antibiotics do kill bacteria, hip replacements do allow people to walk again without pain, broken bones are correctly treated, ruptured appendices removed, fluids correctly replaced after severe trauma, anaesthetics and intensive care do allow people to be operated on, and live. Many people will be kept alive for longer, who would have died in the past.

I would hate people to think that I hate modern western medicine. I love it. I am alive due to western medicine; my appendicitis would have killed me otherwise. My knee works, and my father is still alive, and my mother can still walk due to western medicine.

Because I have so much respect for what western medicine can do when it goes right, I really, really, hate to see it when it goes horribly wrong.

When it is distorted, manipulated and used for the wrong purposes. And when it plucks 'facts' from thin air. I am not going to cover them all here, but I want to give you some idea of how widespread this phenomenon is.

Five a day

This was even more plucked out of the air than a plucked out of the air thing. The reality of '*five portions of fruit and vegetables*' is that it was simply made up at a meeting of fruit and vegetable companies in California in 1991.[140] Even McDonalds were there! Presumably to make sure that the French fry counted. Of course, it still could be true. I await any robust evidence to support it with a baited breath... dum de dum. Nothing so far.

Ever since 'five a day' was coined, there have been various post-rationalisations that people who ate more fruit and vegetables were less likely to get cancer. An observation that should come as no great surprise. Those eating fruit and vegetables were more health conscious, took more exercise, smoked less, drank in moderation, were of higher social class... the usual stuff that makes dietary associations completely unreliable.

Somewhat later on, the health benefits of five portions of fruit and vegetables spread into the world of cardiovascular disease. I am not entirely sure when, how, or why this happened. But it did.

I never really believed it was true, and when I started to dig more deeply into this area the evidence started to melt in front of my eyes. What did anyone mean by five portions of fruit and vegetable in the first place? Was it three portions of vegetables and two of fruit, or could it five of one, and none of the other? Did tomatoes count as a fruit, or a vegetable, or both. What about bananas and coconuts. Coconuts have more saturated fat in them, proportionately, than any steak. Where did avocados fit in?

At first no-one had even made the most perfunctory effort to define what the size of a portion might be. Was it five water melons, or five grapes? Five lentils or five pumpkins. Nor was it remotely clear which vegetables or fruit counted.

More recently, belated attempts have been made to define what a portion of fruit and vegetables might actually be. In the gap, Heinz jumped onto the bandwagon to announce that a big squirt of tomato ketchup can make up one of your five portions of vegetables. I think spaghetti hoops also count. Yes, spaghetti hoops. I saw it on a tin in the supermarket. You could not make this stuff up, unless you wanted to spend the rest of your life in a high security mental hospital.

Although, to be perfectly frank, Heinz claiming that tomato ketchup and spaghetti hoops can make up one of your *five a day*, is no more idiotic than the incoherent nonsense promoted by supporters of the *'five portions.'*

According to the supporters of this dogma it has been decreed that chips (French fries) don't count as a portion of vegetables. Ronald McDonald wasted his time. Indeed, everyone agrees that French fries are almost uniquely unhealthy. How can they possible say this?

A potato is a vegetable is it not? If it is not, what is it? If you fry a potato in vegetable oil then you are effectively frying a vegetable in the oil of other vegetables. So, where do the unique, health damaging properties, creep in – exactly? On the other hand, if you bake a potato it is good for you... ho, hum. Potatoes, the quantum vegetable. It can co-exist as both healthy and unhealthy simultaneously.

Logically, if you go to McDonald's and have a portion of chips fried in vegetable oil, and cover them with a big dollop of tomato ketchup – made from tomatoes – this should really be considered three portions of fruit and vegetables in one big super healthy meal. Should it not?

I know most people would consider this ridiculous. For a number of different reasons McDonald's is viewed today as *the* uniquely unhealthy fast food outlet. It is the poster child for evil corporations that are driving the world to towards obesity and heart disease. The heartless swine. They even rub it in, by demanding that you 'have a nice day.' But not too many of them obviously.

But let me state just again the evidence for eating five portions of fruit or vegetables a day in terms of proven evidence-based benefit is non existent.

When your BMI ≥ 30 , you are obese

Doctors' surgeries all have multi-coloured graphs on the wall with your weight vs. height compared on a charts. You will have seen these charts in many other places as well: health clubs, hospitals, physiotherapy clinics and suchlike.

They consist of a bunch of green squares, orange squares and red squares. Green means you are of healthy weight, orange means overweight, but the scary zone of the red square means that, for your height, you weigh far too much and you are therefore, horror of horrors, obese. Yes, the deadly graph of doom has calculated that you have a BMI greater than, or equal to, thirty.

The validity of this figure is pretty much accepted as gospel. It also appears in all publications on obesity. If your BMI is greater than thirty you are OBESE! You must lose weight, or you will DIE! Yes, yes, blah de blah, we all know this.

But where did the actual figure come from?

Chasing down the genesis of this fact was one of the most difficult challenges I have yet encountered. Normally I am pretty good at hunting down *the* original study, the one that everyone uses to support everything that they subsequently do – even if they are blissfully unaware that this is what they are doing.

I did find that an early National Health and Nutritional Examination Study (NHANES II) study in the United States used a BMI over 32.3 as their 'cut-point' for obesity. And that study ran from 1976 – 1980. NHANES is the biggest, and probably the best, of all nutritional studies.

Which means that the definition of obesity cannot have been set in stone until at least 1980, almost certainly later. In fact, I think it was not until 1995 that it happened. This was when the World Health Organisation finally decreed that obesity was to be defined by a BMI of thirty or more.

The figure itself was agreed at a meeting in Geneva, which generated a long and very boring publication. It stretched to more than six hundred pages. I know, I read it. Somewhere about page four hundred and something I finally came across the passage that I had been hunting for. It was pretty much as I had expected:

"The method used to define BMI cut-off points has been largely arbitrary." [141]

Largely arbitrary. An interesting combination of words. I suppose it sounds a bit better than '*plucked from thin air*'. Or... '*we just made it up, because we felt that we had to say something.*' The world is gripped with terror that so many of us are now obese. I call it the '*largely arbitrary*' epidemic.

As a further slight aside, always be suspicious of nice round figures. Obesity is a BMI > 30, overweight BMI > 25. A high cholesterol level is > 5.0 mmol/L (in the USA 200 mg/dL, which is 5.2 mmol/L) A high blood sugar is > 6.0 mmol/L etc. It is an amazing thing how human measurement systems exactly match the definitions of illness in perfectly simple numbers.

Safe limits for alcohol consumption

Whilst, in most areas, the experts try to cover up the fact that they are just making things up. From time to time the truth emerges.

"The UK government's guidelines on how much it is safe to drink are based on numbers 'plucked out of the air' by a committee that met in 1987. According to The Times newspaper, the limits are not based on any science whatsoever, rather 'a feeling that you had to say something' about what would be a safe drinking level.

"This is all according to Richard Smith, a member of the Royal College of Physicians working party who produced the guidelines. He told the newspaper that doctors were concerned about mounting evidence that heavy long term drinking does cause serious health problems. But that the committee's epidemiologist had acknowledged at the time that there was 'no data', and that 'it's impossible to say what's safe and what isn't.'"

So now you know. When your doctor admonishes you for drinking too much, they are using level V evidence:

LEVELS OF EVIDENCE IN MEDICAL RESEARCH – ADDENDUM
V: A bunch of opinion leaders have been dragged together who have then plucked figures from thin air because they felt they had to say something (See under, WHO definition of obesity).

Once again, with alcohol we have a nice round number. 21 units a week for men is 3 a day. 14 units for women is 2 a day. Amazing, how a unit of alcohol so closely matches definitions of health. Especially amazing as no one has any idea how many units are in anything they consume.

So alcohol recommendations are yes – you've got it – made up. Just as so many of the nanny statements, which try to tell us how to be healthy and live longer, are mostly... made up.

The high cholesterol paradoxes – how one untrue fact leads to another, then another

The greatest number of facts that are just plucked from thin air are the ones that are created in order to support other made up facts. In an earlier chapter I looked at the issue of how medical facts are fashioned simply to 'immunise' against evidence that appears to contradict widely believed hypotheses. Made up things – the entire purpose of which is to support other made up things.

Of all areas of medicine, the cholesterol hypothesis is where we find the greatest number of widely believed 'facts', which were just made up to protect the hypothesis. To remind you of a few:

- Red-wine protects against heart disease;

- Garlic protects against heart disease;

- Excess iron causes heart disease;

- Coffee protects against heart disease;

- Female sex hormones protect against heart disease;

- Antioxidants protect against heart disease... etc., etc.

There are hundreds of these. Even by 1981 a paper managed to identify 261 separate risk factors that either caused, or protected against heart disease. I have no idea how many there now are. Thousands, I would suspect.

Rather than go through them all, which would be exceedingly tedious, I am just going to look at one of these paradoxes/facts in more detail. The reason for choosing this example is to demonstrate how and why this fact came into existence.

The 'fact' is this:

"A low cholesterol level does not cause early death. A low cholesterol is caused by other diseases, and it is the other diseases which actually kill you."

This has been expressed in many different ways, but that is the core of it. The reason why this fact exists is because it has been noted repeatedly that people with very low cholesterol levels, especially elderly people, have a significantly reduced life expectancy.

Now, this does not fit in well with the 'cholesterol hypothesis', which would have us believe that a high cholesterol level is a deadly killer. On the face of it, this is completely contradictory to that widely held idea. Cholesterol can hardly be a killer if you actually live longer when you have more of it in your bloodstream.

When I tell patients that the higher your cholesterol level is, the longer you will live, they look at me as though I am nuts. But it is true, and having a high cholesterol level becomes more and more protective as you get older.

Here is a study published in *The Lancet*: "Cholesterol and all-cause mortality in elderly people from the Honolulu Heart Program: a cohort study."

247

"Only the group with low cholesterol concentration at both examinations [20 years apart] had a significant association with mortality, which was an increased risk of mortality by 64%."[142]

Low cholesterol, mortality increased 64%. I particularly love the final conclusion of this study.

"We have been unable to explain our results. These data cast doubt on the scientific justification for lowering cholesterol to very low concentrations (<4.65 mmol/L) in elderly people."

Oh, would that more researchers were more honest. Although, to be perfectly frank, they didn't really need to explain their findings at all. They could have just said. *'We have found that having a low cholesterol level means that you are 64% more likely die at a younger age.'* How about that, guys. Just the facts, no need for any convoluted opinion, no need for 'further research.'

Further evidence to disprove the *'low cholesterol is caused by underlying diseases hypothesis'* comes from an Austrian study of 150,000 people, done over a period of 15 years. The researchers found that (apart from in younger men, where there was no association), a low cholesterol level was associated with a higher mortality rate in all other groups.

"For the first time, we demonstrate that the low cholesterol effect occurs even among younger respondents, contradicting the previous assessments among cohorts of older people that this is a proxy or marker for frailty occurring with age."[143]

Two very big, very long term studies found exactly the same thing, and there are many more. But there are studies that appear to contradict this. Here, for example is a study published in 1997, which states very clearly.

"Elevated total cholesterol level is a risk factor for death from coronary heart disease in older adults." Corti MC et al: "Clarifying the direct relation between total cholesterol levels and death from coronary heart disease in older persons."[144]

How do two studies find one thing, whilst another finds the opposite. Well, this happens when you re-interpret what you actually find, using the previously mentioned fact: *'A low cholesterol level does not cause early death. A low cholesterol is caused by other diseases, and it is the other diseases which actually kill you.'*

Here is what the Corti study actually found.

248

"Persons [Over 65] with the lowest total cholesterol levels ≤4.15 mmol/L had the highest rate of death from coronary heart disease, whereas those with elevated total cholesterol levels ≥ or = 6.20 mmol/L seemed to have a lower risk for death from coronary heart disease."

Please note the word 'seemed'. Please also note the word in the title of the paper 'clarifying'. These are two words that should not really appear in any scientific paper – ever. Although they do tell exactly what is going to happen next. In this case what is going to happen next is, as follows.

"After adjustment for established risk factors for coronary heart disease and **markers of poor health and exclusion of 44 deaths from coronary heart disease that occurred within the first year,** *elevated total cholesterol levels predicted increased risk for death from coronary heart disease, and the risk for death from coronary heart disease decreased as cholesterol levels decreased."*

Because it is now accepted as a fact that a low cholesterol level is an indicator of poor health, you are allowed to remove deaths from the first year of your study, as these people clearly died from diseases that lowered their cholesterol – rather than the other way round. Once you have done this, along with a bit more statistical jiggery-pokery, you find that, lo and behold, people with *higher* cholesterol levels are more likely to die of heart disease. By using this technique, the conclusions of your study become the exact opposite of what you actually found.

In research, once you re-set your assumptions, you can do almost anything you like with any data. You can remove inconvenient deaths, adjust for any factor you decree to be important, and you can come to the conclusion you wanted in the first place. There is literally, and I mean literally, no end to the data manipulation that is possible within medical research.

I thought you would enjoy a short tale from The Hitchhikers Guide to the Universe at this point:

The Final Proof of the non-Existence of God was proved by a Babel Fish.

Now, it is such a bizarrely improbable coincidence that anything so mind-bogglingly useful could have evolved purely by chance that some have chosen to see it as the final proof of the NON-existence of God. The argument goes something like this:

"I refuse to prove that I exist," says God, "for proof denies faith, and without faith I am nothing."

"But," says Man, "the Babel fish is a dead giveaway, isn't it? It could not have evolved by chance. It proves that You exist, and so therefore, by Your own arguments, You don't. QED"

"Oh dear," says God, "I hadn't thought of that," and promptly vanishes in a puff of logic.

"Oh, that was easy," says Man, and for an encore goes on to prove that black is white (and gets himself killed on the next zebra crossing).

Anyway, here is a challenge for you. Find any study, anywhere, which demonstrates that people with low cholesterol levels live longer than those with higher cholesterol levels. If you believe that you have managed to find such a thing, check for words *seemed*, or *clarifying*, or any other such weasel words. If they are there, you can officially ignore anything that paper says.

The extended 'fact' chain

The example above highlights perhaps the greatest problem with 'facts' that are just plucked from thin air. Or, to be slightly more scientific, facts that are based on low quality data. Once you establish a wrong 'fact' it underpins a chain of interconnected facts that all rely on, and support, each other.

In this situation, things that are clearly nonsense can turn into accepted medical wisdom. For example, people with type 2 diabetes are now advised to eat a high carbohydrate diet. On the face of it this seems utterly ridiculous.

Type 2 diabetes, stripped down to its basics, is a problem with control of blood sugar levels. Carbohydrates are all just forms of sugar, and when we digest them, they are all broken down into simple sugars, such as glucose and fructose. So eating carbohydrates will inevitably raise blood sugar levels.

Logically, therefore, eating carbohydrates would be the worst thing possible for a person with type 2 diabetes to do. How then, did we get to a position where we are telling people with diabetes to effectively eat sugar?

It begins with the diet/heart hypothesis, which is, as I am sure you now know: If you eat fat, specifically saturated fat, your blood cholesterol rises. If your cholesterol rises you are more likely to die from heart disease. This is step one of the process.

Step two happened in the 1970s when it was noted that diabetes was a major risk factor for dying of heart disease. Ergo, diabetics should avoid eating fat, as they are already at a greater risk of heart disease in the first place.

If you believe in the diet/heart hypothesis then the current advice makes perfect sense. Indeed, you couldn't really advise diabetics to do anything else. An extended fact chain, based on the first fact has sent everyone off in a certain direction, as decreed by scientific logic. However, if the hypothesis is wrong, then a high carbohydrate diet will be causing untold damage to diabetics around the world. And that, too, is inevitable.

The super-extended fact chain

The ultimate outcome of bringing fact after fact, study after study together is the, wait for it, drum roll... The meta-analysis. The inarguable crystallisation of all human knowledge on a topic. All hail the mighty meta-analysis.

Whilst you can argue against any single study the meta-analysis is *the* ultimate arguments stopper. At least this is what we are given to believe. But what if the conclusions of that meta-analysis were subject to... to bias? What if they decided to ignore some studies, only include the ones that fit in with dogma? What then?

Surely no-one would ever do this. Would they? Well, of course they would. Here is one such meta-analysis done by the Cholesterol Treatment Triallists Collaboration (CTT). Their hugely influential paper, which underpins guidelines around the world, was called: "Efficacy of cholesterol-lowering therapy in 18 686 people with diabetes in 14 randomised trials of statins: a meta-analysis."

What they found, surprise, surprise, was that statins were enormously effective in preventing heart disease in people with diabetes. They looked at 14 studies which included 18,686 people with type 2 diabetes amongst the various trial populations. They then stripped out the data on people with diabetes. This is called 'data-mining'.

For many reasons, any conclusions from data-mining are far less robust than they would be if the study were specifically set up to look at populations with diabetes in the first place. This is because many of those with diabetes will have other medical conditions e.g. a previous heart attack or stroke. So there is always a danger that you are mixing up any possible effects.

Ideally, if you want to know if statins work in type 2 diabetes then you set up a study in people with type 2 diabetes, and diabetes only. Then you have got rid of 'confounding variables'. Two such studies have been done. The first of these was called ASPEN. The other was called 4D.

251

The researchers putting together the CTT meta-analysis were fully aware of both trials, as they were both mentioned. However, and quite unbelievably, they decided not to include them:

"Since both of these trials reported apparently unpromising results, we considered whether their inclusion would have been likely to change our conclusions."

So they did not include them. Hold on guys. You are doing a meta-analysis of studies done on the use of statins in diabetes and you decided to ignore the only two major studies done specifically in this area. Perhaps, worse than this, the peer reviewers saw no problems with this approach. Well, they couldn't have, or it would not have been published.

I must admit that I find the concept of an *'unpromising result'* in a research paper to be interesting. The entire point of science is an objective search for the truth – at least that is what I understand science to be. Which means that there can be no such thing as a promising, or unpromising result.

Anyone who claims to be a scientist cannot state that a result is *'unpromising'.* In doing so, you have revealed that you are utterly and completely and irrevocably, biased. You have decided what you want to find, and anything that appears to contradict your prejudices – you dismiss as 'unpromising.'

But of course, silly me, it was actually perfectly valid to ignore these two studies. As the authors go on to explain, in a roundabout way:

"Our main conclusions, therefore, are not materially affected by the results of the ASPEN and 4D trials."

True, and also impeccably logical. Their conclusions could not be materially affected by these studies as they DID NOT bother to include them. They also decided to ignore four other statin trials. ALLIANCE, SPARCL, MEGA and GREACE. They had this to say about MEGA:

"In particular, only one of these trials was a primary prevention study (MEGA) and, in view of the small numbers of major vascular events occurring in participants with diabetes in this trial, its inclusion would not be expected to modify our conclusions about the effectiveness of statin treatment in people with diabetes without known vascular disease."

So they didn't actually analyse the data from the MEGA study either, or the other three trials. They just felt that their inclusion would make

252

no difference. This is indeed a wondrous and splendid thing. A meta-analysis, where they don't even bother to analyse data from several major studies. They didn't need to, because they knew that these data would not modify their conclusions.

A meta-analysis, in short, that ignored four major studies, and did not bother to include the only two major studies done specifically on the area of the meta-analysis... bong! Please try again.

Finally, and this time I mean finally, I shall finish this section with an example of how a single study has ended up supporting a vast body of research, and has guided billions of people around the world to alter their diets in response.

This study has underpinned the production and consumption of various low saturated fat foods around the world. It is the key-stone for the vilification of saturated fat, and provides the scientific rationale for multi-billion dollar industry which includes mega- brands such as Flora.

Yet, when you see a press release, such as the one below, you will have not the slightest idea that one trial has done all this:

"A new study provides the first conclusive evidence from randomized clinical trials that people who replace saturated fat in their diet with polyunsaturated fat reduce their risk of coronary heart disease by 19 percent, compared with control groups of people who do not...

"By systematically reviewing a large group of randomized clinical trials and conducting a pooled meta-analysis of these studies, the HSPH [Harvard School of Public Health] team's findings show that increasing the intake of polyunsaturated fats as a replacement for saturated fats could significantly reduce the rate of heart attacks and cardiac deaths in the population. The study appears in the March 23, 2010 issue of the open-access journal PLoS Medicine."[145]

For, once again, we have a meta-analysis. The undisputed highest level of evidence. When you read phrases such as *"the first conclusive evidence from randomized clinical trials"...* you probably think that:

1. This meta-analysis includes new research;

2. This evidence is robust because it is reviewing the 'totality of the evidence';

3. The studies supporting it must be well designed, robust, and of the very highest standard.

Well nothing, and I repeat nothing, could be further from the truth on this one. This press article refers to the Mozaffarian meta-analysis published in 2010. It calls itself a meta-analysis although it only looked at seven different studies. In addition, there was absolutely nothing new here. The most recent of the 7 trials was over 25 years old, and a couple were nearly 50 years old.

So yes, this wasn't a new study at all it was a new analysis of very old studies quite different from a *new study.* But it was a new analysis of very old data.

Not that I have anything against old studies. In fact I tend to trust old studies more than more recent ones as the pressure to produce commercially valuable results was less in those days. However, it should give some pause for thought that a meta-analysis of data which averages 35 years old, can somehow be hailed as new.

Ignoring those points for the moment, the key point here is that the statistical 'significance' of the Mozaffarian analysis relies entirely on a single study. It is the Finnish Mental Hospital Trial. Remove this trial from the meta-analysis and you are left with no statistical significance.

Nothing to say that replacing saturated fat with polyunsaturated fat is beneficial. No reason to eat Flora, no reason for the British Heart Foundation to accept funding from Unilever (who make Flora). No reason to provide dietary advice on replacing butter with margarine. No reason to eat polyunsaturated fats at all.

Whilst you may find this difficult to believe, everything written about the benefits of polyunsaturated fats rests upon the Finnish Mental Hospital Trial. It supports several different meta-analyses and dietary guidelines around the world. A lot of weight for one little study to bear, don't you think.

Therefore, it must be amongst *the* most robust, well-planned and executed of all trials ever done, mustn't it. At this point I was very tempted to say, go look it up yourself and make your own mind up. If there has been any purpose in writing this book it is to make two points. First, *'decide for yourself.'* Secondly, *'don't believe the experts.'*

However, I thought I might give you a few pointers before you start analysing this study for yourself. I would begin by saying that one good thing about having your entire study population confined to two mental hospitals is that you can do what you like with them. Including complete control over what they eat. They most certainly cannot sneak out to the local shops and buy Mars Bars.

So, as dietary studies go, it was very strictly controlled – from the diet side at least. However I was not quite sure how the ethics worked on this. Did all the patients sign up, and agree to take part in a clinical study... every single one? Or did those who refused to take part have to sit in the corner with a dunce's hat on? In fact, I discovered that no-one was asked. The diet was imposed. It was compulsory... jolly good.

Having covered the one obvious strength of this study, here is a starting list of the weaknesses:

- Not randomised;

- Not blinded;

- It had a cross-over design.

The first two points are obvious causes of bias. If you do not have properly randomised population, nor blinding of the participants or observers, this sharply reduces the validity of any study.

In this trial, the patients simply came and went from the hospital, with a loss of about 11% per year of the overall study populations. I cannot think of another clinical study where the patient population studied contained less than 50% of the original study population by the end. When new patients arrived they were simply enrolled into the study, and ended up being the majority. which is a major, major problem.

Using a cross-over design, is perhaps a less obvious issue, but it is a major one. A cross-over design can be a very good idea in some clinical trials. You get a group of people, split them in two, give one half a drug and one half a placebo. Then, half way through, you swap over. This obviously makes your populations perfectly matched, as it is the same population.

This is a good study design if, say, you are looking at the impact on blood-pressure lowering, or pain, or some other non-fatal outcome. Because the patient effectively becomes their own control.

However, if you looking at differences in death rate, a cross-over design is bonkers. If more people die in the first part of the study in one group, you are then crossing over two different, newly unmatched populations. One population will have fewer people in it, for starters.

Clearly, death is not an outcome that you will get two chances to measure after the populations have been switched. Because, to quote from earlier in this book *'You can only die once, of one thing.'* Using a cross-over study design where you are looking at mortality as your primary end-point is just, simply, idiotic.

Researcher: 'Oh look, the people who died in the first part of the study, did not die in the second.'

Second researcher: 'Really, I wonder why that could be.' (Perhaps spoken with a hint of sarcasm).

This problem is further compounded in the area of a dietary study. Whether you believe in the diet-heart hypothesis or not, and I don't, everyone agrees that cardiovascular disease takes many years to develop.

Therefore, changing any diet is extremely unlikely to show any benefit, or harm, over a short period. It is going to take years to have any effect. Which means that, if you put someone on a diet for five years, then change their diet, then they die one week after the change in diet. What group do you include them in? The diet they had been on for five years, or the diet they just started a week ago. In this case they were counted in the diet group they had newly joined. Bong!

Weirdly, the observed benefit in mortality started virtually the day after they switched diet... ho, hum, and how likely is that? Did someone say biased observation.

If we move away from this study for a moment or two, the same researchers who inform us that this trial proved that a very short period of eating a low saturated fat was uniquely beneficial also tell us that you have to eat saturated fats for over 30 years for it to show any harm.

If I may direct you to the *BMJ* once again, and a paper entitled the "Time-lag hypothesis."[146]

As the authors say:

"Summary points:

- *Mortality from ischaemic heart disease in France is about a quarter of that in Britain, but the major risk factors are similar.*

- *Undercertification of ischaemic heart disease in France could account for about 20% of the difference.*

- *The high consumption of alcohol in France, and of red wine in particular, explains little of the difference.*

- *We propose that the difference is due to the time lag between increases in consumption of animal fat and serum cholesterol concentrations and the resulting increase in mortality from heart disease—similar to the recog-*

nised time lag between smoking and lung cancer. Consumption of animal fat and serum cholesterol concentrations increased only recently in France but did so decades ago in Britain.

- *Evidence supports this explanation: mortality from heart disease across countries, including France, correlates strongly with levels of animal fat consumption and serum cholesterol in the past (30 years ago) but only weakly to recent levels. Based on past levels, mortality data for France are not discrepant."*

So, it takes 30 years for eating saturated fat to cause heart disease. It must, otherwise the French – who eat more saturated fat that any other country in Europe – ought to have a very high rate of heart disease. Not a very low rate, as they do.

Of course that paper was published in 1999. So we now can look at the French again many years later. In 1980 the rate of CHD death, in men aged sixty five and under, was 39 (per 100,000 per year). In 2010 it was 26. So, still falling in France guys. Also falling in women.[147]

In France you can eat a high saturated fat diet for 45 years, at the end of which the rate of CHD is still falling. In a Finnish study, you can eat a low saturated fat for less than three years (on average), and it reduces mortality, almost instantly. Something don't add up, guys.

Perhaps Mozaffarian ought to have extended his meta-analysis to include such studies as the Sydney Heart Study.

In February 2013, the *BMJ* published a paper by a team of researchers from the US and Australia who had recovered and analysed the original data from the Sydney Heart Study.

The original Woodhill study involved 458 men, aged 30-59 years old who had recently suffered a coronary event. The men were randomly allocated to one of two groups. The intervention group were instructed to consume a diet of 10% saturated fat and 15% polyunsaturated. The control group were to have 14% saturated and 9% polyunsaturated. Safflower oil and margarine were the substances used to effect this change in the diet group. Safflower oil is a concentrated source of omega-6 linoleic acid and provides no omega-3 PUFAs.

There were 221 men in the diet group and 237 in the control group. There were 39 deaths in the diet group and 28 in the control group. Oops! There were also more deaths from coronary heart disease in the diet group. Oops again.

This was known at the time of the original study, 1978. The authors of the 2013 paper found some data not used in the original report to assess possible *increased* risk of cardiovascular disease.

The researchers concluded that recovery of these missing data "has filled a critical gap in the published literature archive" and that these findings "could have important implications for worldwide dietary advice to substitute omega-6 linoleic acid (or polyunsaturated fatty acids in general) for saturated fatty acids."[148]

In an accompanying editorial, Professor Philip Calder from the University of Southampton says the new analysis of these old data "provides important information about the impact of high intakes of omega 6 PUFAs, in particular linoleic acid, on cardiovascular mortality at a time when there is considerable debate on this question."[149]

Calder said that the findings counter the "saturated fat bad, omega 6 PUFA good" dogma and suggested that the American Heart Association guidelines on omega-6 polyunsaturated fats may be misguided.

Add the Sydney Heart Study to the Mozaffarian meta-analysis and, guess what, there is no statistical significance. Keep the Sydney Heart Study, remove the Finnish Mental Hospital Study, and you will suddenly have a meta-analysis, which proves that polyunsaturated fats increases cardiovascular mortality.

The reality is that meta-analyses really are not the holy grail of medical science. They are not the rock upon which clinical practice should be based. Those who do meta-analyses often decide to include certain studies and not include others for the flimsiest reasons.

As we have seen, you can do a meta-analysis on the benefit of statins in diabetes, and simply ignore the only two major trials done specifically in this area. On the other hand, *all* meta-analyses on the harm of saturated fat, benefit of polyunsaturated fat, include the one statistically significant 'positive' study. This study suffers from such catastrophic scientific weakness that it would be laughed out of court if it had dared to prove the opposite.

The evidence base upon which the gigantic edifice of evidence based medicine rests is, frankly, rotten to the core. Many 'facts' are completely made up. Others rest on observational studies, which are vulnerable to massive bias.

So where does this leave us?

Is there nothing that can be believed anymore, for sure?

I suppose the first step in solving a problem is to admit that there is a problem in the first place. This book, *Doctoring Data*, is my attempt to highlight the fact that we have a massive, massive problem with medical research as it stands today. When the editor of the *NEJM* states (as quoted before):

"It is simply no longer possible to believe much of the clinical research that is published, or to rely on the judgment of trusted physicians or authoritative medical guidelines. I take no pleasure in this conclusion, which I reached slowly and reluctantly over my two decades as an editor of The New England Journal of Medicine."

This should give anyone pause for thought. Richard Smith, who edited the *BMJ* for many years wrote this in a blog recently

"Twenty years ago this week the statistician Doug Altman published an editorial in the BMJ arguing that much medical research was of poor quality and misleading. In his editorial entitled, 'The Scandal of Poor Medical Research,' Altman wrote that much research was 'seriously flawed through the use of inappropriate designs, unrepresentative samples, small samples, incorrect methods of analysis, and faulty interpretation.' Twenty years later I fear that things are not better but worse...

"...'The poor quality of much medical research is widely acknowledged,' wrote Altman, 'yet disturbingly the leaders of the medical profession seem only minimally concerned about the problem and make no apparent efforts to find a solution.'

"Altman's conclusion was: 'We need less research, better research, and research done for the right reasons. Abandoning using the number of publications as a measure of ability would be a start.'

"Sadly, the BMJ could publish this editorial almost unchanged again this week. Small changes might be that ethics committees are now better equipped to detect scientific weakness and more journals employ statisticians. These quality assurance methods don't, however, seem to be working as much of what is published continues to be misleading and of low quality. Indeed, we now understand that the problem doesn't arise from amateurs dabbling in research but rather from career researchers."

Richard Smith finishes this particular blog...

"I reflect on all this in a very personal way. I wasn't shocked when we published Altman's editorial because I'd begun to understand about five years' before that much research was poor. Like Altman I thought that that was mainly be-

259

cause too much medical research was conducted by amateurs. It took me a while to understand that the reasons were deeper. In January 1994 at age 41, when we published Altman's editorial, I had confidence that things would improve. In 2002 I spent eight marvellous weeks in a 15th century palazzo in Venice writing a book on medical journals, the major outlets for medical research, and reached the dismal conclusion that things were badly wrong with journals and the research they published. I wondered after the book was published if I'd struck too sour a note, but now I think it could have been sourer. My confidence that 'things can only get better' has largely drained away, but I'm not a miserable old man. Rather I've come to enjoy observing and cataloguing human imperfections, which is why I read novels and history rather than medical journals."

Sadly, he has just given up the fight. Maybe we all should. The system cannot be fixed? Well, I believe that things can be made better. Once you have read this book and seen the many, many, ways of doctoring data, you can help to make some desperately needed changes. We need to demand that medical research is better than this.

My final word (for now)

This book was going to be a different book. It was going to be about the things I consider to be medical myths. Sunshine is bad for you, saturated fat is terribly unhealthy, salt will kill you, and suchlike. On this basis I was going to call it The Dangerous Book for Grown Ups, shamelessly stealing a title from others. The main theme was going to be that you should just ignore much of what you hear about what is healthy, and what is not. The majority of this information is either irrelevant, or wrong. But I knew that for many, this would feel very dangerous. Going against the mainstream, going against what your doctor tells you, challenging the experts seems scary.

I then thought, why should anyone believe anything that I write. How can Dr Kendrick be right, and all the highly decorated experts be wrong. Well, obviously, they are right about many things. However, when it comes to the area of preventative medicine it seems that every stick that can be grabbed at the wrong end, has been grabbed at the wrong end. Alongside this, experts seem obsessed with simplistic ideas where cause and association are hopelessly muddled. It has become a mess, in part driven by money. Things that are high should be lowered, things that are low should be raised. Yes, we have a drug for that... Kerrching. 'Look for underlying causes? What idiot said that?'

So I decided to try and expose, if that is the right word, how data are produced. How statistics are used to terrify people, or falsely reassure them. Also, what are the drivers for this behaviour? I know I will be attacked for some of the things I have said. That is inevitable. However, that does not matter. What matters is that you, once you have read this book, can understand more clearly how and why data are 'doctored'. You can then understand the headlines more clearly. 'Two sausages a day increase your risk of bowel cancer by 50%. Shock, and horror, and bollocks. You can make the decisions for yourself about what you can and should do to live a longer, healthier and happier life.

That is why I wrote *Doctoring Data*, because knowledge is power.

Acknowledgments and permissions

Cover image: M.C. Escher's "Perfume" © 2014 The M.C. Escher Company – The Netherlands. All rights reserved.www.mcescher.com

Thanks to the Massachusetts Medical Society for permission to reprint the figure on page 70.

Back cover quotation: Dr Marcia Angell. "The Truth about the Drug Companies: How They Deceive Us and What to Do about It." Published by Random House. (August 9, 2005).

References

1   http://www.webmd.com/hypertension-high-blood-pressure/guide/new-low-for-high-blood-pressure

2 Getz L, Kirkengen AL, Hetlevik I et al. "Ethical dilemmas arising from implementation of the European guidelines on cardiovascular disease prevention in clinical practice: A descriptive epidemiological study." Scand J Prim Health Care 22:202-8 (2004).

3 Garland C, et al. "Vitamin D for Cancer Prevention: Global Perspective." Annals of Epidemiology Volume 19, Issue 7 , Pages 468-483 (2009).

4 Michael Baum. "What mammography misses: A breast cancer specialist questions the wisdom of the UK government's screening programme." (2004). http://www.spiked-online.com/Printable/0000000CA382.htm

5 ibid

6 http://www.cancerscreening.nhs.uk/breastscreen/risks.html

7 The BBC. "Campaign warns of drinking 'little too much' alcohol." (February 2012). http://www.bbc.co.uk/news/health-16869618

8 Jeremy Laurance. "Health chief warns: age of safe medicine is ending." The Independent. (March 2012) http://www.independent.co.uk/life-style/health-and-families/health-news/health-chief-warns-age-of-safe-medicine-is-ending-7574579.html

9 The BBC. "'Sausage not steak' increases heart disease risk." (May 2010). http://news.bbc.co.uk/1/hi/8688104.stm

10 The BBC. "Smear tests 'boost cure chances'." (March 2012) http://www.bbc.co.uk/news/health-17221910

11 Huffman MD. "Association or Causation of Sugar Sweetened Beverages and Coronary Heart Disease: Recalling Sir Austin Bradford Hill." Circulation. PMID: 22412071. (2012).

12 David Davis and Max J. Klainer. "Studies in hypertensive heart disease: The incidence of coronary atherosclerosis in cases of essential hypertension." American Heart Journal. (1940). http://www.sciencedirect.com/science/article/pii/S0002870340903441

13 Ioannidis JPA. "Why Most Published Research Findings Are False." PLoS Med 2(8): e124. doi:10.1371/journal.pmed.0020124. (2005.) http://www.plosmedicine.org/article/info%3Adoi%2F10.1371%2Fjournal.pmed.0020124

14 http://www.dailymail.co.uk/health/article-2113986/Red-meat-early-death-study-Eating-regularly-increases-risk-death-heart-disease.html

15 James Alcock. "The Belief Engine." The Committee for Skeptical Inquiry. (1995) http://www.csicop.org/SI/show/belief_engine/

16 Pan A; Sun Qi; Bernstein A; et al. "Red Meat Consumption and Mortality: Results From 2 Prospective Cohort Studies." Arch Intern. Med. (2012).

17 American College of Physicians. Guidelines for Counselling Post-menopausal Women about Preventative Hormone Therapy. Ann Intern Med 117:1038-41. (1992).

18 Writing Group for the Women's Health Initiative Investigators. "Risks and benefits of estrogen plus progestin in healthy postmenopausal women. Principal results from the Women's Health Initiative Randomized Controlled Trial." JAMA. (2002). http://jama.jamanetwork.com/article.aspx?articleid=195120

19 American Medical Network. "A soda a day raises CHD risk by 20%." (2012). http://www.health.am/ab/more/a-soda-a-day-raises-chd-risk-by-20/

20 MRC/BHF Heart Protection Study Press Release. "LIFE-SAVER: World's largest cholesterol-lowering trial reveals massive benefits for high-risk patients." (2001). http://www.ctsu.ox.ac.uk/~hps/pr.shtml

21 Bill Berkrot and Julie Steenhuysen. "Bristol drug cuts death risk in advanced melanoma." Reuters. (June 2010). http://www.reuters.com/article/2010/06/05/cancer-melanoma-bristolmyers-idUSN0218461520100605

22 Medical News Today. "Yervoy (ipilimumab) Turned Down By UK Watchdog." (October 2011). http://www.medicalnewstoday.com/articles/236026.php

23 Black WE, Nease RF Jr, Tosteson AN. "Perceptions of breast cancer risk and screening effectiveness in women younger than 50 years of age." J Natl Cancer Inst. 87 (10): 720-31. (1995).

24 Cancer Research UK (statistics for 2011). http://info.cancerresearchuk.org/cancerstats/types/oral/mortality/

25 Stephen Adams, Medical Correspondent. "Alcohol guidelines 'too high' say doctors." The Telegraph. (January 2013). http://www.telegraph.co.uk/health/healthnews/9774223/Alcohol-guidelines-too-high-say-doctors.html

26 Rostron B. "Alcohol consumption and mortality risks in the USA." Alcohol & Alcoholism. (2012). http://alcalc.oxfordjournals.org/content/47/3/334.long

27 James Shepherd, M.D., et al. "West of Scotland Coronary Prevention Study Group." N Engl J Med. (1995). http://www.cedillapublishing.com/data/Lipid%20sample.pdf

28 Tatu A. Miettinen, MD; et al. Findings From the Scandinavian Simvastatin Survival Study (4S). "Cholesterol-Lowering Therapy in Women and Elderly Patients With Myocardial Infarction or Angina Pectoris." Circulation. (1997). http://circ.ahajournals.org/content/96/12/4211.long

29 Medical Research Council Working Party. "MRC trial of treatment of mild hypertension: principal results." Br Med J (Clin Res Ed). (1985). http://www.ncbi.nlm.nih.gov/pmc/articles/PMC1416260/

30 Odette Wegwarth, PhD; Lisa M. Schwartz, MD, MS; Steven Woloshin, MD; et al. "Do Physicians Understand Cancer Screening Statistics? A National Survey of Primary Care Physicians in the United States." Ann Intern Med. (2012).

31 Roxanne Nelson. "Cancer Screening Data Often Misunderstood By Doctors." Medscape Medical News. (March 2012). http://www.medscape.com/viewarticle/759684?

32 Gardiner Harris. "U.S. Panel Says No to Prostate Screening for Healthy Men." The New York Times. (October 6, 2011). http://www.nytimes.com/2011/10/07/health/07prostate.html?_

33 The BBC. "Smear tests 'boost cure chances'." (March 2012) http://www.bbc.co.uk/news/health-17221910

34 Bengt Andrae, et al. "Screening and cervical cancer cure: population based cohort study." BMJ. (2012). http://www.bmj.com/content/344/bmj.e900

35 Roger Dobson. "Trial stopped early after rosuvastatin found to cut the risk of heart attack and stroke by 44% in healthy people." BMJ. (2008). http://www.bmj.com/content/337/bmj.a2523?

36 Stephen Smith. "Statins cut risk of stroke, heart attack in study." The Boston Globe. (November 10, 2008). http://www.boston.com/news/health/articles/2008/11/10/statins_cut_risk_of_stroke_heart_attack_in_study/ http://www.cancersupportinternational.com/artman/exec/view.cgi?archive=3&num=264

37 From: The New England Journal of Medicine. Paul M Ridker, Eleanor Danielson, Francisco A.H. Fonseca, et al. "Rosuvastatin to Prevent Vascular Events in Men and Women with Elevated C-Reactive Protein." Vol 359., Figure 1. Copyright © (2008). Massachusetts Medical Society. Reprinted with permission from Massachusetts Medical Society. http://www.nejm.org/doi/full/10.1056/NEJMoa0807646

38 Michel de Lorgeril, MD; et al. "Cholesterol Lowering, Cardiovascular Diseases, and the Rosuvastatin-JUPITER ControversyA Critical Reappraisal." Arch Intern Med. (2010). http://archinte.ama-assn.org/cgi/content/full/170/12/1032

39 Sue Hughes. "JUPITER Gets a Battering, But Ridker Fights Back." Theheart.org. (June 29, 2010). http://www.theheart.org/article/1092925.do

40 Bush TL et al. "Estrogen use and all-cause mortality. Preliminary results from the Lipid Research Clinical program follow up study." JAMA. (1983).

41 Inrgid A-L person et al. "Effects of Cocoa extract and Dark Chocolate on Angiotensin-Converting Enzyme and Nitric Oxide in Human Endothelial Cells and Healthy Volunteers." Journal of Cardiovascular Pharmacology. (2010).

42 Heran BS1, Wong MM, Heran IK, Wright JM. "Blood pressure lowering efficacy of angiotensin converting enzyme (ACE) inhibitors for primary hypertension." Cochrane Database Syst Rev. (2008). http://www.ncbi.nlm.nih.gov/pubmed/18843651

43 Robert Lowes. "Red-Wine Researcher Charged With 'Photoshop' Fraud." Theheart. org. (January 13, 2012). http://www.medscape.com/viewarticle/756865

44 http://ec.europa.eu/nuhclaims/

45 Stamler J. "Blood Pressure and high blood pressure aspects of risk." Hypertension (1991).

46 Laura Livesey. "Statins have not been shown to prevent heart disease or heart attacks." The Curious Giraffe. (November 20, 2012).

http://curiousgiraffe.co.uk/2012/11/20/statins-have-not-been-shown-to-prevent-heart-disease-or-heart-attacks/

47 Linda A. Johnson, Associated Press. "Against odds, Lipitor became world's top seller." USA Today. (December 12, 2011). http://usatoday30.usatoday.com/news/health/medical/health/medical/treatments/story/2011-12-28/Against-odds-Lipitor-became-worlds-top-seller/52250720/1

48 Debra S. Echt, M.D., et al and the CAST Investigators. "Mortality and Morbidity in Patients Receiving Encainide, Flecainide, or Placebo — The Cardiac Arrhythmia Suppression Trial". N Engl J Med. (1991). http://www.nejm.org/doi/full/10.1056/NEJM199103213241201

49 Thomas J. Moore. "Deadly Medicine: Why Tens of Thousands of Heart Patients Died in America's Worst Drug Disaster." Simon & Schuster. (1995).

50 http://en.wikipedia.org/wiki/United_States_military_casualties_of_war

51 Michael H. Alderman. "Salt, Blood Pressure, and Human Health." Hypertension. (2000). http://hyper.ahajournals.org/content/36/5/890.full

52 Zosia Kmietowicz. "Antihypertensives are associated with falls in elderly people, study finds." BMJ. (2014). http://www.bmj.com/content/348/bmj.g1736

53 The Action to Control Cardiovascular Risk in Diabetes Study Group. "Effects of Intensive Glucose Lowering in Type 2 Diabetes." N Engl J Med. (2008). http://www.nejm.org/doi/full/10.1056/NEJMoa0802743

54 Nissen SE, and Wolski K. "Effect of rosiglitazone on the risk of myocardial infarction and death from cardiovascular causes." N Engl J Med. (2007).

55 S. Port, A. Garfinkel b, N. Boyle. "There is a non-linear relationship between mortality and blood pressure." Eur Heart J. (2000). http://eurheartj.oxfordjournals.org/content/21/20/1635.refs

56 Wassertheil-Smoller, et al. "Association Between Cardiovascular Outcomes and Antihypertensive Drug Treatment in Older Women." American Medical Association. (2004).

57 Ingela Wiklund, et al and Hot Study Group. "Does Lowering the Blood Pressure Improve the Mood? Quality-of-Life Results from the Hypertension Optimal Treatment (HOT) Study." Blood Pressure. (1997). http://informahealthcare.com/doi/abs/10.3109/08037059709062095?journalCode=blo

58 S.J. Jachuck, et al. "The effect of hypotensive drugs on the quality of life." Managing Hypertension 2. (1982). http://www.ncbi.nlm.nih.gov/pmc/articles/PMC1971011/pdf/jroyalcgprac00086-0041.pdf

59 M. R. Law, et al. "Use of blood pressure lowering drugs in the prevention of cardiovascular disease: meta-analysis of 147 randomised trials in the context of expectations from prospective epidemiological studies." BMJ. (2009). http://www.bmj.com/content/338/bmj.b1665

60 Kelley Colihan. "Taking Statin Drugs Leads to "Modest, but Significant" Drop in Blood Pressure, Study Shows." WebMD Health News. (April 11, 2008). http://www.webmd.com/hypertension-high-blood-pressure/news/20080411/statins-lower-blood-pressure

61 "Drugs of Choice in the Treatment of Hypertension (Part 2)." Therapeutics Letter Issue 8. (Jul - Aug 1995). http://www.ti.ubc.ca/newsletter/drugs-choice-treatment-hypertension-part-2

62 Psaty, Bruce M et al. "Health outcomes associated with antihypertensive therapies used as first line agents. A systematic review and meta-analysis." JAMA. (1997). http://www.ncbi.nlm.nih.gov/pubmed/9042847

63 Francis GS. "Ace inhibition in cardiovascular disease." N Engl J Med. (2000). http://www.ncbi.nlm.nih.gov/pubmed/10639547

64 Avalos EE, et al. "Is dairy product consumption associated with the incidence of CHD?" Public Health Nutr. (2012).

65 Flegal KM, et al. "Excess deaths associated with underweight, overweight, and obesity." JAMA. (2005). http://www.ncbi.nlm.nih.gov/pubmed/15840860

66 http://en.wikipedia.org/wiki/Overweight

67 Lenz M, Richter T,Mühlhauser I, 'The Morbidity and Mortality Associated With

Overweight and Obesity in Adulthood A Systematic Review." Dtsch Arztebl Int. (2009).

68 Orpana H, Berthelot J-M, Kaplam M et al. "BMI and Mortality: Results From a National Longitudinal Study of Canadian Adults." Obesity. (2010). http://onlinelibrary.wiley.com/doi/10.1038/oby.2009.191/full

69 Fred Southwick. "Opinion: Academia Suppresses Creativity. By discouraging change, universities are stunting scientific innovation, leadership, and growth." The Scientist. (May 9, 2012). http://the-scientist.com/2012/05/09/opinion-academia-suppresses-creativity/

70 http://www.duesberg.com/

71 Jeanne Bergman. "Newsweek Exposes Duesberg's Psychopathology." for AIDStruth. org. (14 December, 2009). http://www.serkadis.com/health/26406

72 Dr Malcolm Kendrick. "Blog post: The backlash begins." (November 11, 2013). http://drmalcolmkendrick.org/2013/11/11/the-backlash-begins/

73 Iona Heath. "Overdiagnosis: when good intentions meet vested interests." BMJ. (October 25, 2013). http://www.bmj.com/content/347/bmj.f6361

74 Richard Horton. "Genetically modified food: consternation, confusion, and crack-up." Med J Aust. (2000). https://www.mja.com.au/journal/2000/172/4/genetically-modified-food-consternation-confusion-and-crack (On open view here): http://www.ncbi.nlm.nih.gov/pmc/articles/PMC2688014/

75 Simon Frantz. "From the following article: Pharma's year of trouble and strife." Nature Reviews Drug Discovery 5, 7-9. (January 2006). http://www.nature.com/nrd/journal/v5/n1/box/nrd1944_BX3.html

76 http://www.abc.net.au/science/news/health/HealthRepublish_124166.htm

David L Sackett. "The sins of expertness and a proposal for redemption." BMJ. (May 6, 2000). http://www.bmj.com/content/320/7244/1283.1

77 Dr Marcia Angell. "The Truth about the Drug Companies: How They Deceive Us and What to Do about It." Published by Random House. (August 9, 2005).

78 Richard Smith. "Classical peer review: an empty gun." Breast Cancer Res. (2010). http://www.ncbi.nlm.nih.gov/pmc/articles/PMC3005733/

79 Richard Smith. " Medical Journals Are an Extension of the Marketing Arm of Pharmaceutical Companies." Public Library of Science. (May 17, 2005). http://www.plosmedicine.org/article/info:doi/10.1371/journal.pmed.0020138

80 John Abramson and Barbara Starfield. "The Effect of Conflict of Interest on Biomedical Research and Clinical Practice Guidelines: Can We Trust the Evidence in Evidence-Based Medicine?" Journal of the American Board of Family Medicine. (September–October 2005).

81 Susan Jeffrey. "ALLHAT lipid-lowering trial shows no benefit from pravastatin." Theheart.org. (December 17, 2002). http://www.theheart.org/article/263333.do

82 ibid

83 Howard Wolinsky. "Disease mongering and drug marketing." EMBO Rep. (Jul 2005). http://www.ncbi.nlm.nih.gov/pmc/articles/PMC1369125/

84 Peter C Gøtzsche. "Deadly Medicines and Organised Crime: How big pharma has corrupted healthcare." Published by Radcliffe Publishing Ltd. (August 21, 2013).

85 Dr Malcolm Kendrick. "Blog post: What is your statin-by date?" (November 19, 2013). http://drmalcolmkendrick.org/2013/11/19/what-is-your-statin-by-date/

86 Salynn Boyles. "Study Shows Actos Lowers Risk of Developing Diabetes in People With Prediabetes." WebMD Health News. (March 23, 2011). http://www.medicinenet.com/script/main/art.asp?articlekey=141161

87 http://www.news.com.au/lifestyle/health/pharmacy-guild-to-be-fat-cops-checking-weight-and-peoples-health/story-fneuzlbd-1226820930087

88 http://www.ncbi.nlm.nih.gov/pubmedhealth/behindtheheadlines/news/2014-06-10-one-in-three-adults-in-england-has-prediabetes/   http://bmjopen.bmj.com/content/4/6/e005002.full

89 http://www.nhs.uk/news/2009/12December/Pages/H1N1-swine-flu-virus-death-rate.aspx

90 Letter from BMJ Editor in Chief, Fiona Godlee, to John Bell, Roche Board member. "Tamiflu correspondence with Roche." BMJ. (October 2012). http://www.bmj.com/tamiflu/roche/rr/611576

Troy Brown. "Tamiflu Efficacy, Safety in Doubt, Says BMJ." Medscape Medical News. (November 14, 2012). http://www.medscape.com/viewarticle/774548

91 Kate L Mandeville, et al. "Academics and competing interests in H1N1 influenza media reporting." J Epidemiol Community Health. (2013). http://jech.bmj.com/content/early/2013/10/30/jech-2013-203128.full

92 John Geddes, Peter Szatmari, and David Streiner. "The worm turns: publication bias and trial registers revisited." Evid Based Mental Health. (2004). http://ebmh.bmj.com/content/7/4/98.full

93 Wayne Kondro and Barb Sibbald. "Drug company experts advised staff to withhold data about SSRI use in children." CMAJ. (Mar 2, 2004). http://www.ncbi.nlm.nih.gov/pmc/articles/PMC343848/

94 Katie Thomas and Michael S. Schmidt. "Glaxo Agrees to Pay $3 Billion in Fraud Settlement." The New York Times. (July 2, 2012). http://www.nytimes.com/2012/07/03/business/glaxosmithkline-agrees-to-pay-3-billion-in-fraud-settlement.html

95 Maia Szalavitz. "How Drug Companies Distort Science: Q&A with Ben Goldacre." Time Magazine. (February 28, 2013). http://healthland.time.com/2013/02/28/how-drug-companies-distort-science-qa-with-ben-goldacre/

96 Dr Marcia Angell. "The Truth about the Drug Companies: How They Deceive Us and What to Do about It." Published by Random House. (August 9, 2005).

97 http://www.kolonline.com/

98 KOL Management Solutions. March 2011. http://www.kolonline.com/pdf/FirstWord_KOL%20Mgmt%20Solutions_March%202011.pdf

99 National Heart, Lung & Blood Institute. "ATP III Update 2004: Implications of Recent Clinical Trials for the ATP III Guidelines Updates and Disclosures." (2004). http://www.nhlbi.nih.gov/guidelines/cholesterol/atp3upd04_disclose.htm

100 Silverman E. "Worst Practice? Senate Probes NPR Host's Firm." Pharmalot. (November 21, 2008). Originally published on: http://www.pharmalot.com/2008/11/worst-practice-senate-probe-npr-hosts-firm/ Archive available from: http://www.healthyskepticism.org/global/library/item/17470

101 McLean B. A bitter pill for one Merck critic. Fortune Magazine. (November 29, 2004). http://archive.fortune.com/magazines/fortune/fortune_archive/2004/12/13/8214229/index.htm

102 http://en.wikipedia.org/wiki/Eric_Topol

103 Correction. "Unreported Financial Disclosures in: Association of LDL Cholesterol, Non–HDL Cholesterol, and Apolipoprotein B Levels With Risk of Cardiovascular Events Among Patients Treated With Statins: A Meta-analysis." JAMA. (April 25, 2012). http://jama.jamanetwork.com/article.aspx?articleid=1148176

104 Curtis Brainard. "NYT's reporter explains why it's so hard to "sniff out" conflict of interest." Columbia Journalism Review: The Observatory. (March 27, 2008). http://www.cjr.org/the_observatory/ct_scans_and_tobacco_funding.php?page=all

105 Iona Heath. "Independent statins review panel report. Supporting Documentation SP21: CTSU Grants May 2014." BMJ. (August 1, 2014). http://www.bmj.com/content/independent-statins-review-panel-report-0 (SP21)

106 Science Media Centre. "Expert reaction to decision not to retract two BMJ articles on statins. (August 2, 2014). http://www.sciencemediacentre.org/expert-reaction-to-decision-not-to-retract-two-bmj-articles-on-statins/

107 Patrick A. Malone. "New Health Care Law Will Expose Drug Manufacturers' Gifts to Doctors." DC Medical Malpractice & Patient Safety Blog. (March 29, 2010). http://www.protectpatientsblog.com/2010/03/new_health_care_law_will_expos.html

108 Sidney M. Wolfe. "Patient Advocacy Groups and Drug Company Funding." Public Citizen. (April 2011). http://www.citizen.org/Page.aspx?pid=4898

109 http://www.alzheimers.org.uk/site/scripts/documents_info.php?documentID=302

110 The pharmaceutical industry now controls NHS policy – hoorah http://drmalcolmkendrick.org/2014/02/12/the-pharmaceutical-industry-now-controls-nhs-policy-hoorah/

111 Fiona Godlee. "Say no to the free lunch." BMJ. (April 14, 2005). http://www.bmj.com/content/330/7496/0.8

112 Peter C Gøtzsche. "Deadly Medicines and Organised Crime: How big pharma has corrupted healthcare." Published by Radcliffe Publishing Ltd. (August 21, 2013).

113 Richard Smith. " Medical Journals Are an Extension of the Marketing Arm of Pharmaceutical Companies." Public Library of Science. (May 17, 2005). http://www.plosmedicine.org/article/info:doi/10.1371/journal.pmed.0020138

114 Dr Melissa Walton-Shirley. "ACC 2012 opening session: To Epcot with Braunwald." Theheart.org. (March 24, 2012). http://www.medscape.com/viewarticle/802049

115 Blog Praise of Folly. "AZT: A Medicine from Hell." (October 1998). http://www.sidasante.com/azt/debazt2.htm#AZT:%20A%20Medicine%20from%20Hell

116 Margaret A. Fischl et al and The AZT Collaborative Working Group. "The Efficacy of Azidothymidine (AZT) in the Treatment of Patients with AIDS and AIDS-Related Complex." N Engl J Med. (1987). http://www.nejm.org/doi/full/10.1056/NEJM198707233170401

117 John Lauritsen. "AZT on trial." Virusmyth homepage. (October 19, 1987). http://www.virusmyth.com/aids/hiv/jltrial.htm

118 Blog Praise of Folly. "AZT: A Medicine from Hell." (October 1998). http://www.sidasante.com/azt/debazt2.htm#AZT:%20A%20Medicine%20from%20Hell

Concorde Coordinating Committee. "Concorde: MRC/ANRS randomised double-blind controlled trial of immediate and deferred zidovudine in symptom-free HIV infection". The Lancet. (1994) http://www.thelancet.com/journals/lancet/article/PIIS0140-6736%2894%2990006-X/abstract

119 Bernard Lown. "A Maverick's Lonely Path in Cardiology (Essay 28). (March 10, 2012). http://bernardlown.wordpress.com/2012/03/10/mavericks-lonely-path-in-cardiology/

120 Garfinkel D, Zur-Gil S and Ben-Israel J. "The war against polypharmacy: a new cost-effective geriatric-palliative approach for improving drug therapy in disabled elderly people." Isr Med Assoc J. (2007). http://www.ncbi.nlm.nih.gov/pubmed/17642388

121 Doron Garfinkel and Derelie Mangin. "Feasibility Study of a Systematic Approach for Discontinuation of Multiple Medications in Older Adults: Addressing Polypharmacy." Arch Intern Med. (2010).

122 Dr Des Spence. "Kill the QOF." BMJ. (March 6, 2013). http://www.bmj.com/content/346/bmj.f1498

123 http://www.dailymail.co.uk/news/article-2378434/Mystery-sudden-rise-elder-ly-death-rates-600-people-dying-week-2013-compared-past-years.html

124 David R. Flum et al. "Early Mortality Among Medicare Beneficiaries Undergoing Bariatric Surgical Procedures." JAMA. (2005). http://jama.jamanetwork.com/article.aspx?articleid=201707

125 Abdal Raheem et al. "Bariatric surgery complications leading to small bowel transplant: a report of 4 cases." J Parenter Enteral Nutr. (2014). http://www.ncbi.nlm.nih.gov/pubmed/23636011

126 Gwenaëlle Douaud et al. "Preventing Alzheimer's disease-related gray matter atrophy by B-vitamin treatment." Proc Natl Acad Sci U S A. (June 4, 2013). http://www.ncbi.nlm.nih.gov/pmc/articles/PMC3677457/

127 George Davey Smith. "Commentary: Behind the Broad Street pump: aetiology, epidemiology and prevention of cholera in mid-19th century Britain." International Journal of Epidemiology. (2002). http://ije.oxfordjournals.org/content/31/5/920.full.pdf

128 Madison Leigh Rose. "John Snow and the Cholera Myth." (August 27, 2012). http://madisonleighrose.wordpress.com/2012/08/27/john-snow-and-the-cholera-myth/

129 Mark Grant. "Galen on Food and Diet." Published by Routledge. (2000).

130 Andy Coghlan. "Family win $1.5 million in autism-vaccine payout." New Scientist. (13 September, 2010). http://www.newscientist.com/blogs/shortsharpscience/2010/09/family-win-15-million-in-autis.html

131 Centers for Disease Control and Prevention. "CDC statement on narcolepsy following Pandemrix influenza vaccination in Europe." (February 26, 20913). http://www.cdc.gov/vaccinesafety/Concerns/h1n1_narcolepsy_pandemrix.html

132 "Vaccine damages, Vaccine injuries and adverse effects of vaccinations in babies, infants, children and adults." (2010). http://www.vaccineinjury.info/vaccine-damages-in-general.html

133 Booth NE, Myhill S, McLaren-Howard J. "Mitochondrial dysfunction and the pathophysiology of Myalgic Encephalomyelitis/Chronic Fatigue Syndrome (ME/CFS)." Int J

Clin Exp Med. (2012). http://www.ncbi.nlm.nih.gov/pubmed/22837795

134 http://www.skepticat.org/2010/04/dr-myhill/

135 Michael O'Riordan. "Statin-Induced Myopathy Reflects Structural Muscle Damage, New Study Shows." Theheart.org. (July 07, 2009) http://www.theheart.org/article/984185.do

136 There are a number of different definitions of levels of evidence in medical research. (http://www.patient.co.uk/doctor/different-levels-of-evidence) Patricia B. Burns, Rod J. Rohrich and Kevin C. Chung. "The Levels of Evidence and their role in Evidence-Based Medicine." Plast Reconstr Surg. (2012) http://www.ncbi.nlm.nih.gov/pmc/articles/PMC3124652/

137 Dr Malcolm Kendrick. "Blog post: Guidelines kill 800,000." (January 20, 2014). http://drmalcolmkendrick.org/2014/01/20/guidelines-kill-800000/

138 Larry Husten. "Medicine Or Mass Murder? Guideline Based on Discredited Research May Have Caused 800,000 Deaths In Europe Over The Last 5 Years." Forbes Magazine. (January 15, 2014). http://www.forbes.com/sites/larryhusten/2014/01/15/medicine-or-mass-murder-guideline-based-on-discredited-research-may-have-caused-800000-deaths-in-europe-over-the-last-5-years/

139 http://www.escardio.org/guidelines-surveys/esc-guidelines/Documents/DOI-PERIOP.pdf

140 Zoe Harcombe. Blog post: Five a day: The truth." (March 11, 2012). http://www.zoeharcombe.com/2012/03/five-a-day-the-truth/

141 National Institutes of Health Consensus Development Panel on the Health Implications of Obesity. Health implications of obesity. National Institutes of Health Consensus Development Conference Statement. Ann Intern Med 1985;103:1073-77. http://www.ncbi.nlm.nih.gov/pubmed/4062128

142 Schatz IJ et al. "Cholesterol and all-cause mortality in elderly people from the Honolulu Heart Program: a cohort study." The Lancet. (2001). http://www.ncbi.nlm.nih.gov/pubmed/11502313

143 Ulmer H et al. "Why Eve is not Adam: prospective follow-up in 149650 women and men of cholesterol and other risk factors related to cardiovascular and all-cause mortality." J Womens Health (Larchmt). (2004). http://www.ncbi.nlm.nih.gov/pubmed/15006277

144 Corti MC et al. "Clarifying the direct relation between total cholesterol levels and death from coronary heart disease in older persons." Ann Intern Med. (1997). http://www.ncbi.nlm.nih.gov/pubmed/9148647

145 Harvard School of Public Health. "Replacing saturated fat with polyunsaturated fat may cut heart disease risk." Science Daily. (March 23, 2010). http://www.sciencedaily.com/releases/2010/03/100322211831.htm

146 Malcolm Law and Nicholas Wald. "Why heart disease mortality is low in France: the time lag explanation." BMJ. (May 29, 1999). http://www.ncbi.nlm.nih.gov/pmc/articles/PMC1115846/

147 European Heart Network and European Society of Cardiology. "European Cardiovascular Disease Statistics 2012 edition." (September 2012). http://www.bhf.org.uk/plugins/PublicationsSearchResults/DownloadFile.

aspx?docid=352b602f-e110-4fca-89ec-a24229e7a1c0&version=-1&title=European+C
ardiovascular+Disease+Statistics+2012&resource=HS2012EC

148 Christopher E Ramsden et al. "Use of dietary linoleic acid for secondary prevention of coronary heart disease and death: evaluation of recovered data from the Sydney Diet Heart Study and updated meta-analysis." BMJ. (February 5, 2013). http://www.bmj.com/content/346/bmj.e8707

149 Editorial. "Study raises questions about dietary fats and heart disease guidance." BMJ. (February 4, 2013). http://www.bmj.com/press-releases/2013/02/04/study-raises-questions-about-dietary-fats-and-heart-disease-guidance

INDEX

C

CABG 195, 196, 197, 198, 199, 200;

Calder, Philip 258;

Cancer - Breast 11, 12, 13, 14, 15, 41, 42, 50, 122, 181, 189, 194, 231, 265, 266;

Cancer screening 9, 12, 13, 15, 20, 23, 42, 57, 58, 60, 61, 62, 63, 64, 65, 68, 122, 181, 227;

Cancer - Skin 7, 11;

Cardiovascular disease 45, 71, 72, 77, 82, 92, 96, 102, 106, 111, 112, 115, 130, 149, 231, 243, 256, 258, 265, 268, 281;

Cervical cancer 20, 61, 62, 63, 64, 65, 66, 67, 267;

Charlton, Bruce 25, 134;

Cholera 219, 220, 272;

Cholesterol xiii, 7, 8, 9, 12, 29, 30, 34, 35, 51, 52, 53, 71, 74, 78, 80, 81, 82, 83, 84, 85, 86, 88, 91, 92, 94, 95, 113, 125, 126, 130, 137, 138, 139, 147, 148, 149, 151, 159, 160, 161, 165, 166, 172, 177, 181, 201, 213, 217, 235, 245, 246, 247, 248, 249, 250, 251, 256, 257, 266, 267, 270, 271, 273, 281;

Chronic Fatigue Syndrom (CFS) xiii, 29, 53, 138, 159, 165, 166, 172, 228, 229, 230, 231, 232, 233, 247, 251, 266, 267, 271, 272, 273, 281;

Circulatory System xiii, 29, 53, 101, 138, 159, 165, 166, 172, 221, 222, 247, 251, 266, 267, 271, 273, 281;

Cleveland clinic 69, 164, 165, 167, 168, 169;

Climate change 25, 80;

Clinical Trial Service Unit (CTSU) 168, 169, 271;

Cochrane 87, 113, 122, 152, 161, 162, 267;

Cole, Graham 240;

Collins, Rory 34, 35, 169;

Coronary artery bypass 195, 197;

Coronary Heart Disease (CHD) 21, 32, 51, 78, 111, 113, 114, 115, 117, 118, 145, 197, 199, 200, 257, 265, 266, 268;

Creatinine Kinase (CK) 232, 233;

Crystallotherapy 234;

D

Daily Mail 27, 205;

DECREASE 240, 241;

Deep vein thrombosis (DVT) 100, 187;

Department of Health 9, 10, 151, 159, 200, 223;

Diabetes 8, 9, 11, 20, 30, 35, 81, 97, 113, 115, 118, 143, 147, 149, 150, 151, 158, 173, 174, 203, 226, 234, 250, 251, 252, 258, 268, 270;

Diabetes UK 173, 174;

Diagnostic and Statistical Manual of Mental Disorders 147, 148;

Duesberg, Peter 123;

E

Einstein, Albert 132, 184, 201;

European Heart Journal 104, 240;

European Society of Cardiology (ESC) 8, 239, 242;

F

Familial Hypercholesterolaemia (FH) 130;

FDA 163, 170;

Feldman, Stanley 16, 17;

Female Sexual Arousal Disorder (FSAD) 146, 147;

Finnish Mental Hospital 254, 258;

France 138, 200, 256, 257, 273;

Francis, Clare 229;

Francis, Darrel 240;

French paradox 83;

G

Galen 221, 222, 272;

Gastric bypass 207;

Gastric ulcers 134;

General Medical Council (GMC) 130, 131, 231;

Geneva Declaration 154;

Germany 124, 225, 228;

277

Medical Research Council (MRC) 54, 55, 56, 103, 104, 106, 107, 113, 266, 272;
MEGA 252;
Meijer, Melchior 125, 129;
Meta-analysis 87, 120, 166, 238, 240, 251, 252, 253, 254, 257, 258, 268, 271, 274;
Metabolic Syndrome 147;
Miasma (infection) 220, 221;
Mintze, Dan 159;
Mintzes, Barbara 171;
Mitochondria 223, 230, 231;
MONICA 85;
Montaigne, Michel de 61;
Mortality 15, 17, 27, 28, 30, 32, 48, 49, 50, 51, 52, 53, 56, 57, 58, 60, 69, 70, 71, 72, 73, 74, 75, 78, 94, 96, 101, 104, 113, 119, 120, 121, 132, 145, 186, 187, 191, 198, 202, 203, 209, 210, 219, 247, 248, 256, 257, 258, 265, 266, 267, 268, 269, 272, 273;
Murray, John 175, 176;
Myalgic Encephalomyelitis (ME) 228, 229, 230, 231, 232, 233, 272;
Myhill, Sarah 231, 232;
Myocardial infarction 32, 55, 185, 186, 195, 268;

N

Narcolepsy 224, 272;
National Cholesterol Education Programme (NCEP) 159, 160, 161, 162;
National Health Service (NHS) 10, 15, 37, 38, 39, 40, 174, 175, 271;
National Heart, Lung, and Blood Institute (NHLBI) 159;
National Institute for Clinical Excellence (NICE) 38, 39, 40, 47, 138, 281;
National Institutes of Health (NIH) 159, 161;
New England Journal of Medicine (NEJM) 85, 97, 130, 139, 140, 150, 157, 178, 200, 240, 259, 267;
New York 220;

Nissen, Steven 69, 71, 74, 167, 168;
Nobel Prize 112, 124, 135, 137, 158, 236;
Null hypothesis 53, 54, 107;
Nutmeg 220, 221;

O

Obesity 9, 10, 118, 119, 120, 121, 132, 147, 201, 207, 208, 210, 244, 245, 246, 268, 269, 273;
Osteoporosis 201;

P

Pandemrix 224, 272;
Paroxetine 155, 156;
Pasternak, Richard C. 145, 146;
Pasteur, Louis 219;
Paxil 155, 164;
Paxman, Jeremy 117;
Peer review 133, 134, 240, 241, 269;
Placebo 23, 35, 52, 54, 55, 56, 69, 70, 71, 72, 73, 74, 75, 103, 105, 106, 107, 116, 180, 191, 192, 193, 255, 267;
Plank, Max 132, 136;
PLoS Medicine 178, 253;
Poldermans, Don 131, 241, 242;
Polling, Hannah 223, 232;
Polypharmacy 195, 200, 202, 203, 205, 272;
Polypill 114;
Popper, Karl 84, 145, 184;
Pre-diabetes 150, 151;
Pre-hypertension 8, 112, 150;
PROSPER 162;
Prostate cancer 11, 15, 58, 59, 60, 61, 62;
Publication bias 154, 270;
Pulsed Electromagnetic Therapy (PET) 235;

Q

Quality Adjusted Life Year (QALY) 39, 40, 47;
Quality Outcome Framework (QoF) 195, 200, 201, 202, 204, 205;

R

Rath, Matthias 192;
Ravnskov, Uffe. Dr xiii, 74, 126, 130, 139, 180;
Rennie, Drummond 140;
Resveratrol 88, 89;
Ridker, Paul 69, 73, 130, 166, 267;
Rosch, Paul 180;

S

Sackett, David 135, 136, 269;
Salt 7, 12, 98, 181, 261, 268;
Saturated fat 7, 29, 80, 84, 85, 139, 243, 250, 253, 254, 256, 257, 258, 261, 273;
Semmelweis, Ignaz 219;
Seroxat 155;
Simvastatin 51, 201, 266;
Skin Cancer 7, 11;
Smear test 20, 21, 61, 66;
Smith, Richard 143, 246, 259, 269, 271;
Snow, John 219, 220, 236, 272;
Solar system 214, 216;
Southwick, Fred 122, 269;
SPARCL 252;
Specialised Healthcare Alliance (SHCA) 174, 175;
Spence, Des 204, 272;
SSRIs 155;
Statins 34, 35, 37, 38, 39, 40, 52, 56, 69, 71, 72, 74, 95, 109, 110, 112, 125, 126, 130, 131, 138, 145, 146, 149, 160, 161, 162, 163, 165, 166, 167, 181, 227, 232, 233, 251, 252, 258, 267, 268, 271;
Stent 198;
Stroke 7, 8, 19, 32, 35, 42, 46, 47, 48, 55, 68, 69, 71, 73, 74, 92, 96, 99, 100, 101, 102, 103, 106, 107, 111, 112, 113, 114, 115, 148, 201, 251, 267;
Sunshine Act, the 158, 169, 239;
Surrogate end-points 91, 93, 94, 116;
Sydney Heart Study 257, 258;
Syndrome X 147;
Systolic blood pressure (SBP) 8, 92, 99, 105, 107;

T

Tamiflu 151, 152, 153, 270;
Taubes, Gary 180, 181;
Thalidomide 111;
The Poverty of Historicism 184;
Thiamine (B1) 210;
Thucydides 79;
Tired All The Time (TATT) 234;
Tolstoy, Leo 80;
Topol, Eric 164, 165, 167, 271;
Trotter, Wilfred 79, 141, 213;
Twain, Mark 214;

U

US Navy 217;

V

Vaccination 151, 223, 224, 225, 226, 228, 231, 272;
Viagra 111, 112;
Vioxx 164, 165;
Vitamin D 11, 265;

W

Wakefield, Andrew 226, 227, 228, 231, 232;
Warren, Robin 134, 135, 236;
Wegener's hypothesis 184;
West of Scotland Coronary Prevention Study (WOSCOPS) 50, 162;
Widowmaker 196, 199;
Women's Health Initiative (WHI) 31, 79, 83;
World Health Organisation (WHO) 19, 85, 245, 246;

X

X-ray 15, 196;

Y

Yeats, W.B. 214;

About the author

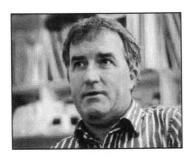

Dr Kendrick graduated from medical school in Aberdeen and trained as a General Practitioner in Scotland. After ten years he split his time between General Practice and education. On the doctor side, Malcolm currently lives and works in Cheshire in General Practice, Intermediate Care and Out of Hours. On the education side, Malcolm set up the on-line educational system for the European Society of Cardiology, working with the European Commission and also set up the first website for the National Institute for Clinical Excellence (NICE) in the UK.

Malcolm is an original member of the Centre for Evidence Based Medicine in Oxford and of The International Network of Cholesterol Sceptics (THINCS). The latter comprises a group of scientists, doctors and researchers who share the belief that cholesterol does not cause cardiovascular disease.

This is the field of medicine for which Malcolm is best known. His long term interest in the epidemiology of cardiovascular disease has resulted in many publications in journals such as the *BMJ*, *Medical Hypotheses*, *Pulse* and *PharmacoEconomics*. His breadth and depth of expertise in this area led to his election to Who's Who in 2009.

The Great Cholesterol Con was the book that firmly placed Malcolm on the world stage of the 'diet-cholesterol-heart' hypothesis and his army of followers are eagerly awaiting his next bout of wit and wisdom. Malcolm blogs at drmalcolmkendrick.org and lectures by invitation.

Married with two children and two cats, Malcolm would like more people to challenge the status quo, and never just accept the party line. He likes to ski, golf, sail, play squash, walk in the hills and drink... not necessarily in that order.

21528997R00167

Made in the USA
San Bernardino, CA
24 May 2015